HOW TO INCREASE YOUR
STAND UP PADDLING
PERFORMANCE

First published in 2015 by Suzie Trains Maui

© 2015 Suzie Cooney

ISBN-13: 978-1517158156
ISBN-10: 151715815X

Author: Suzie Cooney
Managing Editor: Katie Elzer-Peters
Cover Design: Brooke Foreman Scarborough
Production & Layout: Nathan Bauer

HOW TO INCREASE YOUR
STAND UP PADDLING PERFORMANCE

BEGINNER TO ELITE

BY SUZIE COONEY

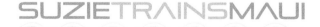

SUZIETRAINSMAUI

With Gratitude

I'd like to express my sincerest thanks to those who helped me bring this book to life. I am beyond grateful for the support that flows my way each and everyday and I want to give special recognition to those extra special few who have

. . . *encouraged* me: Justin Edwards, Bill Hofmann, Mike Adrian, Gregg Leion, Jon Ham, Salma Ansari, Michelle Wagner, Simone Reddingius, John Beausang, Casey Fukuda, Matthew Murasko, Synneve Andrena, Cathy Gillis, Stephan Ross, Joel Edwards, Kevin and Jenney V., Mahalo.

. . . *inspire* me: Kathy Shipman, Jeremy Riggs, Dave Kalama, Ralf Sifford, Peggy King, Milton Kalani Martinson, Kody Kerbox, Kai Lenny, Loch Eggers, Bill Boyum, Andrea Moller, Manca Notar, Devin Blish, Jen Fuller, Johnny Kessel and many more.

. . . been supportive and loving when I was cross-eyed, absent from fun, and chained to my desk for days and nights on end, my boyfriend Tommy Callan.

. . . and finally to the most amazing, patient mentor, my "book trainer" and talented editor, Katie Elzer-Peters of The Garden of Words, LLC, and my awesome production artist, Nathan Bauer of Yellow Cow Design & Media.

HOW TO INCREASE YOUR
STAND UP PADDLING PERFORMANCE
FROM BEGINNER TO ELITE

CHAPTER 1
Equipment Check: Gear Matters

- Does your gear match your style of paddling?
- Is it time to upgrade your SUP equipment?
- Learn why every board shape has a purpose.
- Board/Paddle Talk: Terms you should know.
- Suzie's favorite SUP gear & accessories.

There are two main pieces of equipment necessary to standup paddling: the board and the paddle. How do you know you have the right board and paddle for the job? More importantly, do you understand why you need a specific board or paddle for different conditions?

If you're just getting into stand up paddling you may have noticed the plethora of different shapes, lengths, and constructions of available paddleboards. There are now even inflatable boards for those who live in big cities or like to literally pack and go. Whether you SUP surf small or large waves, cruise and explore on lakes and flat water, or are into downwind surfing, there's a specific board to suit your purpose.

If you're a seasoned paddler you may find yourself with an average of three to six boards—one for every condition. Of course you'll also have a few different paddles, too.

On Maui, I proudly admit, there have been times I've had more boards than I had shoes! I had boards for small waves, big waves, cruising, coaching, and downwinders. I also have multiple paddles, each suited for different conditions and different board lengths. Some allow me a faster cadence, while others help me pull more water.

Before you get started on the exercises and techniques in this book, do an equipment check and make sure that your boards and paddles match up with the type of paddling activities you enjoy most.

BOARDS

Having board knowledge, from the different types of construction to the different purposes of various stand up paddleboards, will help you in selecting a board that allows you to accomplish your desires and goals. There's epoxy, carbon, hollow construction, wood and foam sandwich composites, molded EPS and so on. Again, we're talking about stepping up your total SUP performance so it's time to learn as much as possible, from A-Z.

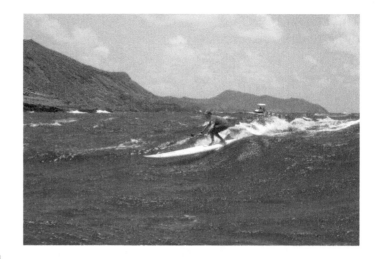

Here's a great shot of downwind champ and my coach, Jeremy Riggs, dialing in his downwind board, surfing some amazing bumps. Notice how long and narrow this board is. It also has an on-board steering system.

BOARD TALK

Here are a few key paddleboard-related terms that you should know about when you start thinking about an upgrade or addition to your quiver. Some of these terms cross over from other board sports such as surfing and windsurfing.

Quiver: Having more than three boards.

Length: This is the distance from nose to tail on the board. It's really important select the right length to the SUP activity you're doing. SUP boards range from 6ft up to 18ft long. You will match your skill set, height, and weight with the length of the board you're considering. Size matters! Surf SUP boards are usually on the shorter side. Cruising and more recreational types are between10 feet and 12 feet and then open ocean, channel crossing, and distance SUP boards are usually 12 feet up to 18 feet+. I've seen custom boards that are longer than 18 feet.

Width: This is the distance from rail to rail. (Side to side.) As important as the length, the width of the board also impacts your performance. Some boards are 20 inches wide (fairly narrow) but can be up to 35 inches (really wide). Too narrow and you could struggle, too wide and you might paddle in slow circles. The width measurement is taken at the widest part of the board.

Thickness: This could also be called the "height" of the board. SUP boards are definitely heavier than thinner surfboards but some are incredibly light. Lighter is nice but it can also mean more fragile and it will for sure cost more. Thickness can range from 3 ½ inches up to 6 inches or more. If you're a heavier person, a thicker board will float you better (see Volume). If you're on the lighter side, you may get away with a thinner board. Some people like wafer-thin boards. Those require more skill and balance.

Volume: SUP board volume is also referred to as number of total liters the board displaces in the water. There are many formulas for calculating your ideal weight to board volume ratio. The end result of all of them is board stability and floatability. This can be critical when designing a high performance custom board. It's a helpful spec if you're on the heavier side and you want the board to float you without being a dead log. Or, if you're lighter, you can manage less board volume to gain board speed. SUP board liters can range from 92 liters up to 275 liters.

Board rocker: Rocker is the angle or curve of the board from nose to tail. There is **nose** rocker and **tail** rocker in paddleboards. It can vary in different degrees of scooping to flat to even turned under. Similar to surf boards, a more turned up nose rocker on a SUP board can make the board turn easier for catching waves. Low rocker offers more board surface area on the water, which is great for flat water racing.

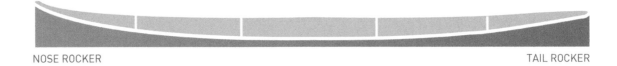

NOSE ROCKER   TAIL ROCKER

RAIL TYPES

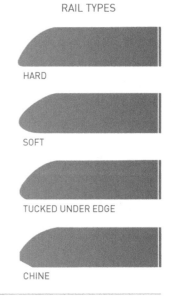

Tail rocker, also known as tail kick, makes a board lift, stick, or be loose for catching more waves. If your SUP board has more tail rocker it may be easier to control but it could also slow you down.

Rail line: This is the template or outline of your SUP board. It can be rounder or narrower with the purpose of more turns for wave riding or faster sprinting and speed.

Rails: The rails of your SUP board are the edges of the board. They run from the nose to the tail. They are usually thinner in the nose (except in some flatwater boards with thick hull designs), thicker in the middle, and tapered down

HARD

SOFT

TUCKED UNDER EDGE

CHINE

in the tail. The angle of the rail or curve can be more round to almost squaring off on some tail designs.

A "softer" (rounder) rail is nice for wave riding. A hard rail angle will bite and help you control the board for flat water racing and help you increase speed. I've had boards that are combinations with a sort of displacement nose and soft tail rails that finish off with a harder edge at the tail. These boards worked amazingly well for flat water and open ocean downwinders.

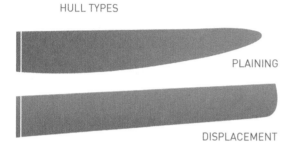

HULL TYPES

PLAINING

DISPLACEMENT

Displacement hull: This refers to the shape of the nose of the board. Think of a canoe or bow of a ship when you think displacement hull for a SUP board. If you need to punch through a bump or if you want maximum speed cutting through a body of water, this shape of nose can offer that. You can also visualize this nose to be a couple inches taller and pointier, allowing for the water to glide on either side of the nose versus the board gliding on top of the water and the water moving underneath it.

Planing hull: This is the most common board nose shape and what most people experience paddling during their first attempt at SUP. This board shape is usually wider and more stable. Most all SUP surfboards have this shape of hull or nose.

Recessed deck: On this type of board, the deck of the board (top of board) where you stand is sunk below the top rails of the board. Decks can be recessed by several inches or just one or two. The recessed part usually begins just above the handle (about 6 to 12 inches) and extends towards the tail, eventually rising up.

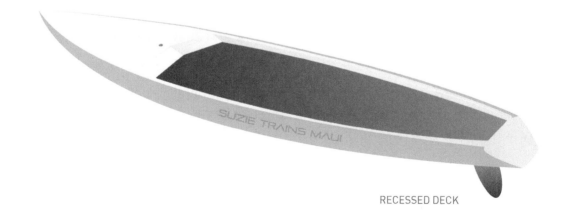

RECESSED DECK

Some recessed decks extend all the way out to the edge of the tail. These decks are popular and offer stability while you're driving hard from flat to chop.

Tails: Like the nose, the tail of your SUP board matters, particularly as your skills increase. The shape of the tail of the board determines how you'll turn or hold a line on the water. The tail shape impacts the way the SUP board stabilizes during a glide.

Like surfboards, the tail of a SUP board responds to the water that is pushed towards the back of the board as it seeks the line of release. I personally think the tail is super critical when it comes to upping your total performance. So get as geeked out as you like.

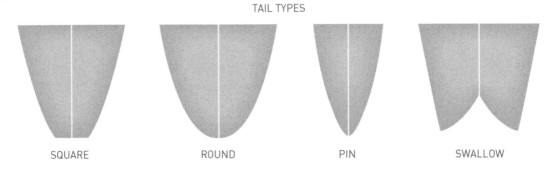

TAIL TYPES

SQUARE   ROUND   PIN   SWALLOW

The most common type of tail is the **rounded tail.** This is tail makes the board easier to plane and creates a smoother turn. Boards with rounded tails are more stable.

Then comes the v-shaped **pin tail**, which is better-suited for surfing larger waves and taking steeper drops. This tail won't throw you as fast and holds on during deeper turns. It won't work as well on smaller waves and is, overall, less stable. I've seen some downwind boards with nice pin tails that allow you track and maneuver at higher speeds.

There are also a few **swallow tails** out there are fun on smaller waves. The two points that make an upside down W bite a bit more and attack a larger surface area on the wave.

Finally, there's the **square tail.** Boards that have a square tail usually have less rocker overall and are great for quick pivot turns while racing. This type of tail offers stability at higher speeds.

SELECTING A BOARD

I would say this part of gear selection can be intimidating for some. It's a bit overwhelming these days as the sport grows in so many different dimensions, offering endless styles of boards for every paddling preferences. Over the years boards have gotten lighter, have better handle slots indented for ease of carrying, and some even have cool loops that also carry your paddles. If you can increase your breadth of knowledge about boards, as a consumer it will help your overall outcome, and that's the name of the game here.

I recommend investing in a board you can manage on your own, and that means lifting it for transport, not just being able to paddle it well. If you can't lift the board you paddle then you need to come train with me! I strongly believe in this. If you have to wheel your board over a long distance to the water that's fine too.

When buying a new board, learn everything you can about conditions in your area or region. If you're lake racing or entering paddle surf contests, look around on the breaks and lakes and see what types and styles of boards the better paddlers are riding. It's a good bet that they've tested a few boards and know what works well.

Taking the world by storm are now the ever-popular inflatable boards that are pretty amazing. Their integrity and stiffness offers anyone the opportunity to travel the world and paddle on lakes, down rivers or even on the waves. Some come with pumps that you hook up to your car battery and some come with pumps that are self-charged and ready to go.

Inflatables are all the rage and should not be overlooked and can be used as a great training board as well. They are durable and now are raced around the world.

I've seen students and people I've coached that have really strong paddling skills, excellent balance, and incredible footwork that were being held back by their gear—as in, the gear wasn't advanced enough.

I've also seen the opposite—people that have an expensive, nice paddle and board that they hadn't quite grown into yet.

I've seen people struggling with speed, paddle cadence, or catching waves and it's not always their lack of strength or board time. I've seen people of different size proportions sink their board so much they could barely paddle. I've also witnessed those with shorter arms and height struggle to extend their reach to their full potential because their boards are too wide therefore prohibiting their maximum paddle stroke.

A mismatch in gear cannot always be overcome by technique and training.

If you want to be fast, your board needs to be fast. If you want to carve up the waves, you need a snappy, more responsive board. If you're racing down rivers in Colorado you need fast and durable.

Downwind paddleboards are a unique animal unto their own requiring the right tail shape, length and nose rocker. Some even have built in steering systems with a rudder to accommodate regular and goofy footers that help you navigate side chop and help you maximize glides. They are incredible and range in sizes from 14 feet up to 18 feet. Some are hollow custom and some are production. In photo below I'm on my 16 foot hollow carbon F16. I love this board. They are custom made for Maliko downwinders.

If you're considering a channel crossing in your future, I highly recommend a board with a rudder and steering system because they will help you conserve energy—as much as 40 percent, and will allow you to go much faster against side winds and strong currents. They'll help you catch many more bumps when the action heats up, too.

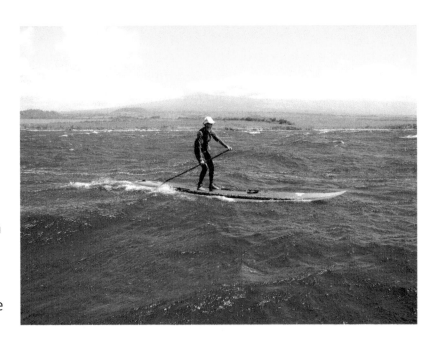

You may also consider getting a custom board made for you. You get to select all of the characteristics of the board in its final design. It's a cool experience, but it's expensive. Before you order, you need to know exactly the shape and style you are seeking. It's always an awesome feeling to hop on YOUR new, custom baby made to your height, weight and ability.

So, bottom line, when you want to be the best you can be, it's okay to have more than one board. If you've got space and are wiling to adjust your finances a bit, you can have it all. Just don't forget to save enough money to eat! You'll need to eat well for the next chapter.

PADDLES

If you are going to step up your total performance for stand up paddling, you need to make sure you have a decent paddle. I'm not saying break the bank, but at least start with a paddle that suits your style. This will also help you avoid early fatigue and possible injury. There are many great brands, including KIALOA, Quickblade, Naish, and more.

Some argue that the paddle is the most important piece of your SUP gear. I would agree, to some point. Using the right one, or few, can make a huge difference in your paddle experience. Don't spend all your date money, but for sure make the investment on a good one that fits you because, after all, we are talking about stepping up your SUP performance.

There are three parts to a paddle and the shape, size, and construction of each part determines the function, comfort, and durability of the paddle. When selecting a paddle you'll look at the shaft, blade, and handle.

Opinions and theories are all over the water with opinions all over the map about which type of paddle shaft, width of blade, degree and/or pitch angle of blade, bend of shaft, and so forth, is best. I have seen the SUP paddle evolve and have tried many. I've also experimented with different paddle weights and different combinations of all of the variables above. Because many of you will be advancing to the next level while working through this book, take the time to learn everything you can and test-drive a few different paddles.

PARTS OF THE PADDLE

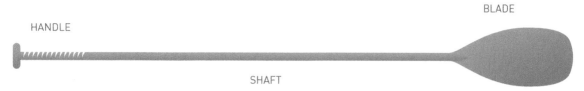

Handle: The top of the paddle. You grip the handle with your top hand. Even handles are getting tricked out and custom-made. Some people will pop out the actual handle of the paddle it comes with and slide in a handle that may have finger grooves or a more rounded shape. Some also have a nice, padded neoprene top that helps reduce hand fatigue.

Some more recreational-type paddles often come with a harder, resin plastic type of handle to reduce costs. The paddle shaft and blade may be decent but the handle can hurt your hand. If you find yourself switching out the handle for a different feeling handle or material, be sure the diameter of the base matches that of the shaft. It's best to get help from a local shop when doing so. They'll be best at gluing and taping the handle for a secure fit.

Paddle shaft: Stem of paddle from the handle to the insertion of the blade.

The paddle shaft can be constructed from different types of materials, including aluminum, carbon, light wood, and fiberglass. Some have a blended construction such as fiberglass and carbon, offering a nice all around paddle without breaking the bank.

Some shafts are tapered, narrowest at the top where the shaft meets the handle, getting fatter at the insertion point where the shaft meets the blade. I've also used paddles with oval-shaped shafts, which can lead to more comfort if your hand is on the smaller side. It's really cool how some of these paddles feel.

I personally like the average-sized diameter shaft so I can feel like I'm pulling something substantial. The paddles with skinnier shafts that are targeted towards women don't give me that powerful pull that I like to feel. However, on the flip side, when I need to paddle a faster cadence I do like somewhat of a skinnier shaft.

A closing note on SUP paddle shafts: With your new strength gains after reading this book, you will learn to use your entire body to advance your board forward, not just your paddle. You will also start noticing certain flex patterns in the shaft.

For example, when I'm SUP surfing, I want my paddle shaft to be a little more flexible to help me brace on a wave. That is in comparison to my downwind paddle shaft, which is much stiffer and full carbon, in order to deliver huge blasts of power to help me catch all the bumps and maximize my glides.

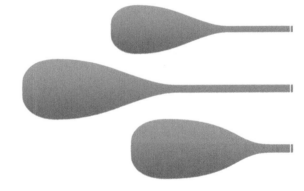

Blade: The blade is the part of the paddle that enters the water.

Tall, wide, dihedral, v-drive, double dihedral; just to name a few different blade options. You'll select the blade shape and size based on your level and preference.

TOP: WIDER BLADE AT BOTTOM: POWER STROKES GOOD FOR DOWNWINDERS
MIDDLE: WAVE/TOURING SHAPE
BOTTOM: DIHEDRAL, LOW ENTRY LESS PITCH: FOR RACING

How to Increase Your Stand Up Paddling Performance

Widths and shapes of paddle blades will vary, as will construction, just as with boards.

As you become a stronger paddler you'll start noticing the way the blade enters (catches) and exits the water and how it can affect your stroke. This is not to be taken lightly. Your start and finish can depend on it.

Your speed and cadence for flat water and sprinting is dependent upon your ability to bring that paddle as fast as possible to the next stroke. So finding a blade that is designed for that is key.

If you're paddle surfing you need quick power in 2-3 strokes or you might miss that wave. What's going to be the best blade choice for you? A fatter, teardrop shaped blade. Also you don't want the shaft of your paddle too short or too long. If it's too short your lower back will kill you and if it's too long you'll risk injuring your shoulder, and, it's almost a guarantee that your traps and rhomboids will revolt. When deciding the right size for your paddle it's best to have a little bend at the elbow, but not too much.

For downwind paddling, I'm always on the lookout for a blade that gives me all the power I can handle without sacrificing my shoulder endurance. I want a blade that I can handle for the times I may have to grind it out when the wind drops, but one that also gives me a thrust of power to catch the bumps.

The length of your paddle for downwinding will be a bit longer than that of your cruising length paddle, and for sure longer than the length of your surfing paddle. Now some of you may debate this, but think, if you've got a few more feet of board out there, such as a 14 foot or 16 foot board, you have more to reach for. A short stubby paddle will not help.

I'm not going to say exactly how long your paddle for downwinding should be, but your hand should almost reach the handle and your elbow may have only a very slight bend. I used two paddles during the M20 (Molokai to Oahu channel crossing). I used my longer paddle for the crossing and shorter one as I approached the finish to Oahu. The side wind and faster cadence forced me into a different stroke. It was really nice to be able to ramp up my actual paddling stroke.

When I'm coaching I try to get students immediately connected to the "feeling" of how the blade behaves. I make small suggestions on how it should feel and how they can maximize the surface area of the blade. I also make sure that when they paddle, the paddle is fully entering the water and not just what I call "ticking" the top of water, thereby underutilizing the full power of the blade.

In relation to this, when you're upgrading to a nicer paddle, you want to be able to understand what the term "purchase" is. That refers to the amount of power you can grab from the blade when the blade is properly buried into the water. That initial entry matters, as does the shape of your blade, to get the maximum purchase power based on the conditions presented.

Some blade shapes will be square, some will be teardrop and others may have a huge flair at the bottom. If you look closely at a rack of paddles and really start examining them closely, you'll also see the pitch or angle of the blade can vary from almost flat, all the way to having a serious bend upwards. Most angles range from 10-13 degrees.

BLADE PITCH AND ANGLES

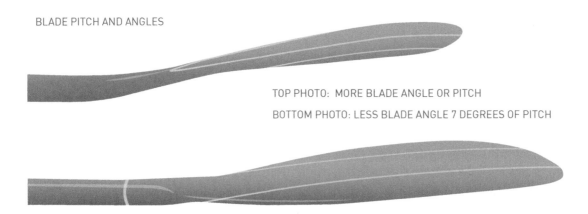

TOP PHOTO: MORE BLADE ANGLE OR PITCH

BOTTOM PHOTO: LESS BLADE ANGLE 7 DEGREES OF PITCH

Personally I've tried a few and I like the blades that are not quite flat but offer a small pitch. I feel like I'm able to get such a nice press through the water. Now, this is interesting. I tried a paddle with a blade that had an extreme pitch in angle and immediately, two things happened, I swear I felt the blade wobble and cavitate. I also lost so much power it felt like I was paddling with a toothpick.

Don't get overwhelmed, but the more you know, the better paddler you're going to be. It's truly amazing the different theories and research that has gone into making the paddles especially for stand up paddling more efficient. I really appreciate the beauty of a nice paddle and all the efforts I can see and feel in the performance.

PICKING A PADDLE

Different conditions call for different paddles. As with board shapes, paddle trends are always changing. There are lots of references about how to be properly fitted for paddle length, but one key point is often overlooked, and that's blade width. While some companies tout this or that, it boils down to what's most comfortable without losing performance and power. If you get the chance, try and demo before buying.

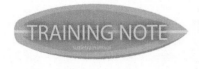

As the sport grows and more and more people advance their paddling, one of the most common complaints I hear time and time again, is about shoulder fatigue and rotator cuff challenges that can often be caused by pulling too much of a blade and paddle. Learn more about how to avoid shoulder problems in Chapter 10 when I talk about how to avoid shoulder injuries.

Some paddles and shafts are made from a composite (combination of different materials) and offer good performance and durability. You will more than likely get a little more weight with this, which could inhibit your top performance. However, on the flip side of that blade, I've actually used a paddle once that was too light and I couldn't get the power I felt I needed. It was the strangest feeling.

Generally speaking, here are some rules of thumb to keep in mind when selecting a paddle: (personal preferences will vary)

Surfing: Flexible shaft, shorter length
Cruising: Combo fiberglass/carbon is fine, average blade width
Downwinding: Full carbon, longer length is most efficient
Flat water sprint racing: Stiff carbon, taller blade shape, shorter length

Traveling with a paddle, especially your expensive carbon race paddle, can be an issue, as the airlines don't often treat them with the care you hope. The upside is that now you can get pretty nice three-piece paddles that break down for ease of travel, from plane to subway

One style of paddle that's trending but again may not be the "best" in power output or stiffness are adjustable paddles. I have a few and use them for teaching and I really like having options sometimes on a downwinder if I find myself in a section that is serious side chop. I love having the option to slide the side down an inch or two. You can also get these in full carbon that are pretty cool.

Also, as conditions changes from head wind to side wind, to downwind, adjustable paddles are all the rage and are also referred to as varios. These have really come a long way and I use them often from the surf to downwind training.

For example, there are a lot of secret spots on Maui that require me to paddle quite the distance just to get to the breaking reef. Typically I like my paddle surfing paddles to be a bit on the shorter side. But, if I have to paddle far I could burn a lot of energy doing so and my lower back might get sore.

What you sacrifice in power output, you gain in flexibility and overall comfort during your paddle.

As you get stronger and become more aware of your own capabilities, you'll be able to fine-tune your selection for all conditions and styles of paddling. I'll talk more about this in Chapter 10 when I discuss how, for example, paddling with a blade that's too wide can lead to early shoulder fatigue. You'll also learn how the length of your paddle can lower your power output, so be sure to check that out.

Test as many paddles as possible and stick to carbon if you can afford it. This will offer the best performance from beginning to end. In the end, you'll probably end up with a minimum of two paddles.

SUZIE'S SUP GEAR & ACCESSORY FAVORITES

With every sport there is gear. I love gear of all of kinds but especially the gear and accessories that I use to complete, not my outfits, but to complete my SUP performance.

I'm grateful to partner with companies that provide me with the best equipment, including fuel, eye protection, skin protection, training equipment, and paddling tops.

First mention goes to **Indo Board Balance Trainer**. You will notice they are a huge contributor to this book and my life and they have been in my corner for many years. I'm grateful for their friendship and support and for the way their gear has transformed not only my clients' SUP performance, but mine too. I could not do what I do without Indo Board Balance Trainer. A big Mahalo to Hunter, Chip and Gette. Check out the gear and get training today.

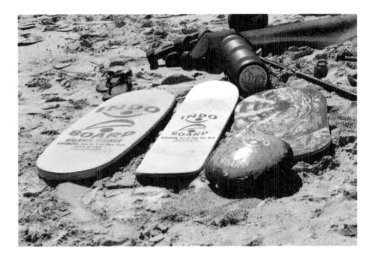

Next on board, my long time friends at **Kaenon Polarized Eyewear**. Besides keeping me stylish and helping me see every bump on the Maliko runs, I love the shades off the water. Kaenon are truly dedicated to the science behind the lens in providing the best in performing technology. The new Soft Kores are the absolute bomb, are super comfortable, and stay on. Great for racing downwind and in the flats.

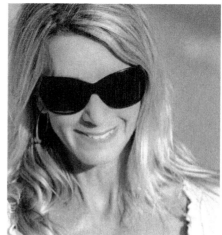

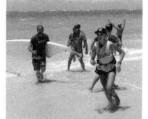

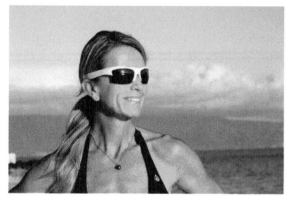

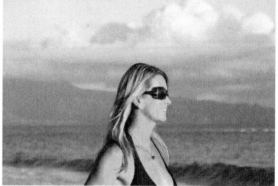

I can't speak highly enough of the performance gear that **BLUESMITHS** provides me in paddling tops. They are Maui tested and made from a unique hydrophobic fabric that offers the best in sun protection. Water beads up and runs off, which keeps you dry. I feel so much more confident in my paddling when I'm in Bluesmiths, especially on the huge, scary days during a Maliko run. When it's just me and the massive swells and these tops and allow me to move with comfort while I tackle the water.

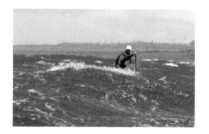

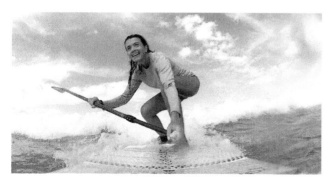

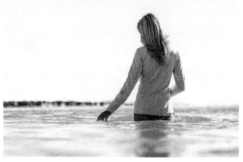

I love **Pocketfuel Naturals** to fuel me during my downwinders. This is real super-food that gets into your bloodstream quickly and delivers real nutrition when you

need it most. The butter blends are my favorites because they are easy to digest AND it tastes like I'm eating chocolate nutella. What could be better? I don't get sick, spike, or crash when I use Pocketfuel Naturals, and I could not do my channel crossings without them.

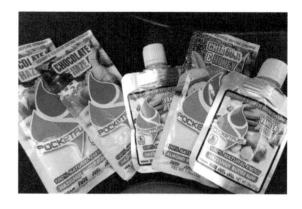

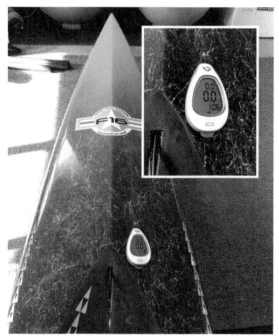

Another great training and motivation tool is called the **Makai**. It's manufactured by **Velocitek** can be used for downwind or SUP racing. This is a cool GPS and Doppler shift driven device easily mounts on any board to track your real time speed, distance, and time. Its big readout makes it easier to use than looking at my wrist device and it keeps me moving.

Learn more about how it can be best used in Chapter 11 which is all about downwind paddling.

And finally, the most important, is my skin protection. I am so thankful to have discovered the best organic sunscreen that does not hurt the ocean, the fish, or me! **RAWElements USA** is all natural and stays on. It never runs in my eyes. The founder is a lifeguard captain and understands the damage the sun can do. This is the best-rated organic sunscreen on the market and it works.

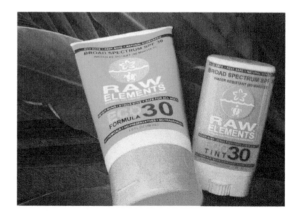

CHAPTER 2
How *NOT* to Be an All Arm SUP Paddler: It Begins with the Core

- What is the core and how does it relate to stand up paddling?
- What does it really mean to engage your core as you paddle?
- How to find your "real core power" with each stroke.
- My top five progressive exercises to build the foundation of your stand up paddling.
- Ab Exercises: AB-solutely we must train the abs.

In this chapter I'm going to help you strengthen your core in order to take you to a higher level of stand up paddling. This chapter includes my top five best exercises. We'll specifically target ways to transfer the power from your core to the water. You will REALLY notice the difference as you train for paddling in waves, flat water, and for downwinders. Without a strong core your paddling will suffer, or, at the very least, won't improve.

WHAT IS THE CORE AND HOW DOES IT RELATE TO SUP PERFORMANCE?

Your core can be defined as "all parts of your body excluding the extremities," and is also referred to as the lumbo-pelvic-hip complex. Think of the core as the muscles that help you gain that extra stroke, that extra glide to the finish, or help you get into the next wave. The core connects your arms and legs so they can work together while you paddle.

The core helps you stabilize and balance from the center of your body, out, and you want it to be solid as a rock. For example if you have strong glutes (butt muscles) and lower back muscles, you will feel less stress on the lower half of your body as you brace against the face of a wave or when you go for a cutback. Or, with a strong core, you can outlast your opponent in a distance or sprint race because you will not fatigue as quickly.

Additionally, with a super strong core, your stroke can be extra explosive because you will have the necessary correct, functional body mechanics that create an extra punch while you paddle.

CORE MUSCLES
The muscles of your core include two groups: Major and Minor

Major Core Muscles: pelvic floor muscles, transversus abdominis, multifidus, internal and external obliques, rectus abdominis, erector spinae (sacrospinalis) especially the longissimus thoracis, and the diaphragm.

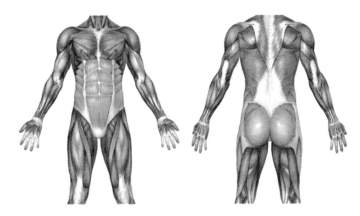

Minor Core Muscles: latissimus dorsi, gluteus maximus, and trapezius.

ENGAGING YOUR CORE DURING STANDUP PADDLING

You have probably read over and over again in many SUP training related articles to "engage your core." I've been writing about this since 2010 so I hope I can explain it best.

If I were paddling next to you and I told you to turn on the power from your obliques *NOW*, you might look at me like I have three heads. Pro SUP athletes say, "okay," and blast away from me. That's what I want for you. I have a specific exercise that will help you turn that on in your brain and in your body.

Let's think about it in terms of a slow motion stroke on the left side. As you're reaching for the nose of your board with the bottom of your left shoulder, your left hip bone is also pointed in that direction, and, of course, your chest should be facing the opposite (right) rail. (If you don't understand this, come out for a lesson with me on Maui or you can SKYPE with me.)

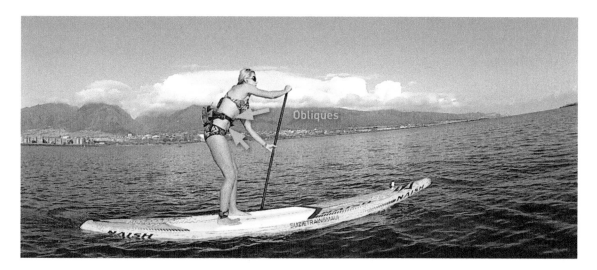

Now you're reaching with your paddle, squaring up the bottom part of the blade and, just at the second your paddle enters the water, BAM! You should contract your deepest left muscles of the core or more specifically, your deep transverse abdominis and the internal oblique first. THEN you can let your hip complex and shoulder complex help you finish the stroke.

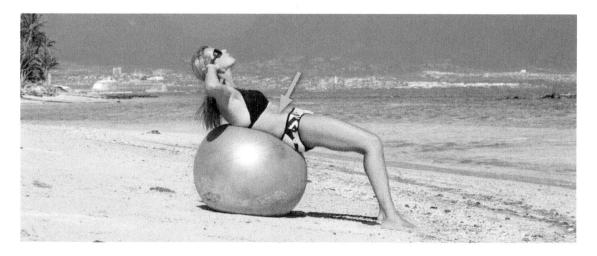

The feeling you should be experiencing when you're engaging and contracting your deep core muscles is the same feeling you get when you do an oblique (or side) crunch on top of a stability ball, and you stop at the top and hold for a second or two.

Think of your core as a constant in your training—not an accessory to your training. It needs to be a huge priority if you want to be faster and stronger. When I say or suggest that it's not a good idea to be an all arm paddler, what I mean is that you shouldn't rely on being super buff in your upper body alone. Sure, that really helps, but if you're too reliant on your big biceps or amazingly sculpted chest, you're missing out on a lot of power.

Include core training in each training session. I recommend doing 2-4 exercises of the core each time you train. The more core exercises you know and can to choose from (called "variables" in your training), the more successful you'll be on the water.

It's like changing conditions. If you're really good at flat water paddling and you only train on flat water and then suddenly you're placed into a different paddling environment, your results could suffer. My point is—don't plateau in any type of training. Mix it up.

HOW TO FIND YOUR "REAL CORE POWER" WITH EACH STROKE

Now that you've got a better understanding of how the core serves your performance as a stand up paddler, let me help you find that real power. To really get a grasp of what I'm about to share here, you'll need to put on your visual visor and imagine every word I say while you're paddling.

It's a beautiful morning on Maui and it's time to head down to the harbor and do some laps. It's just before dawn and there in the parking lot are Kody Kerbox, Conner Baxter, and Kai Lenny, and, of course, Bart DeZwart already putting in some friendly chasing laps.

I'm stoked, because who could ask for more motivation and inspiration than this?

I've got my Garmin charged and my goals set for the morning. I need to get my real core power on— especially when the side winds hit.

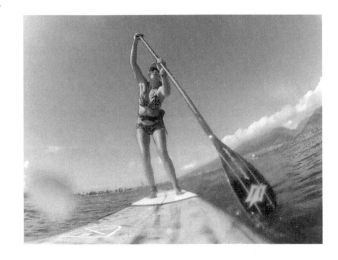

My warm up is going great. I'm paddling nice and easy to buoy number one, about a half a mile away, just inside the mouth of the harbor. I turn left and there's a small, gentle swell that's pushing me but is also pulling me back a little with each stroke.

Warm up over; game on! I look to my left and in the corner of my eye there are the Maui boys full on in their sprint. I think to myself, "Here we go—time to get lapped pretty soon," but I give it my best. I need every ounce of "core" power with every stroke if I've got any chance this morning.

My first thought is to contract the obliques and turn them on for a test. Left on. Right on. I can feel that they are engaged. I'm so aware of this that my shoulders and hips naturally do their thing and I become a smooth paddling machine.

I've gotten so good at this that I can tone down the contraction intensity as necessary. I hope the same is soon true for you. You'll want to work on this kind of control throughout your training and throughout a race or contest. This applies to sprint and distance training too.

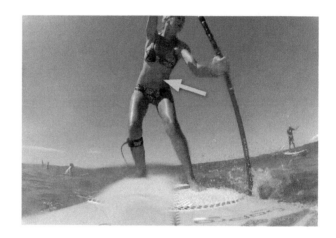

You'll also adjust for the waves. For example, when I see a wave building, as I get myself into a position to catch it I turn on the obliques and REALLY dig in to help me leverage more power to the blade so that I can guarantee that I catch that wave in 2-3 strokes max. If I don't manage that, I usually miss the wave.

CORE EXERCISES

These exercises are challenging. Do your best and progress slowly as so that you keep good form throughout. My suggestion is to incorporate 2-3 of these core exercises into each total body training session. You can progress safely once you've mastered each progression without compensation at any joint extremity. The progressions I list for each exercise start with the least challenging version, working up to the maximum level of difficulty.

Even though some photos are of me barefoot in the sand, I suggest that you wear supportive athletic shoes while training in order get the most out of the following exercises and to assure the best form and outcome.

Have fun!

Exercise 1:
SIMPLE PRONE PLANK WITH PROGRESSIONS

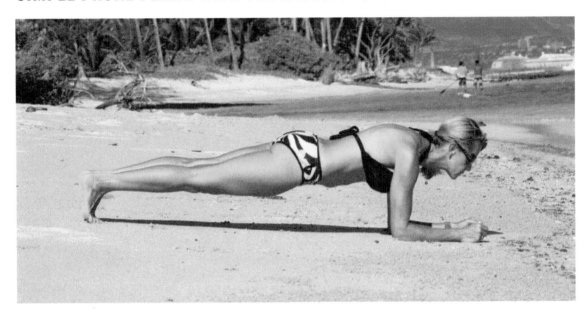

SUGGESTED TRAINING EQUIPMENT
Cushioned floor mat, INDO Board 24" Gigante Cushion, BOSU

SUGGESTED REPS/SETS
1-3 sets, timed increments of 15 seconds, 30 seconds, 45 seconds, 1 minute+

PROGRESSION VARIABLES
Two legs to one, stable surface to unstable surface, forearm plank to push up position

While assuming the prone (face down) position, lie on floor with your feet together and forearms on ground. Your shoulders should be stacked in alignment with your elbows at a 90 degree bend. Do not clasp hands/fingers together.

Lift your entire body off the ground until your back forms a straight line from head to toe while you're resting your weight on your forearms and toes. Draw in your abs (do not hold your breath) toward the front of your spine and *keep breathing*. Imagine squeezing a lemon in front of your spine. Keep your head in a neutral position and don't look up. Try to make sure your butt is not sticking up in the air! Bring it down in alignment so that your back is like a plank of wood. Hence the name.

Hold for 1 -15 seconds, 30 seconds, 45 seconds—working up to one full minute. You may shake like a small earthquake at first, but this is normal. With practice, this will lessen and you'll be rock solid.

PROGRESSION 1

Lift right leg behind you about six inches off the ground, and squeeze the glute of that raised leg. Try holding for 15 seconds then switch to left. Return to plank.

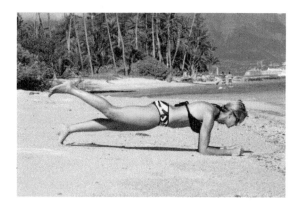

PROGRESSION 2

Next turn the BOSU upside down and assume plank position with hands on the handles to the outside rim. Use a light grip and relax. Extend your legs behind you as you see in photo and same progression, two legs to one. Love this!

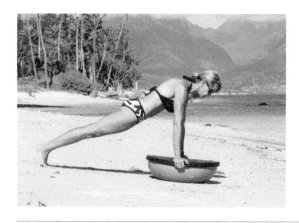 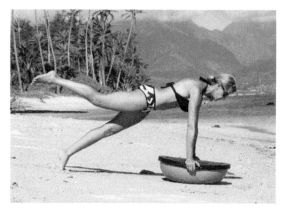

Exercise 2:
ADVANCED PRONE PLANKS WITH PROGRESSIONS

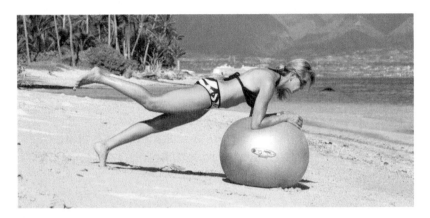

Again, we assume the standard prone plank position but this time we stabilize our forearms on top of an unstable surface. Crazy fun & challenging!

SUGGESTED TRAINING EQUIPMENT
Large stability ball 55-65cm, cushioned floor mat, INDO Board 24" Gigante Cushion, BOSU

SUGGESTED REPS/SETS
1-3 sets, timed increments of 15 seconds, 30 seconds, 45 seconds, 1 minute+

PROGRESSION VARIABLES
The same leg progressions will follow as above, but here change up the arm platforms

PROGRESSION 1

Now that your core is getting stronger, take the stability ball and prepare to assume the standard plank position.

Note: *Firmer inflation equals more speed and instability.*

At first I suggest you have your feet behind you about one foot apart. Continue with the feet progression. Now try brining your feet closer together, then to one leg, feet on BOSU.

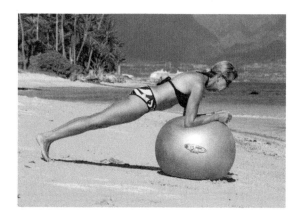
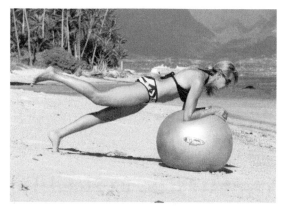
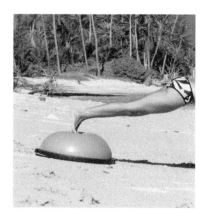
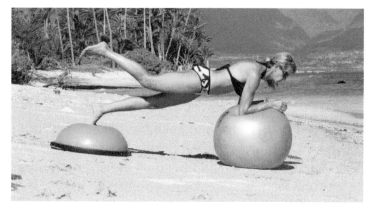

PROGRESSION 2

Crazy advanced

While in the forearm plank atop the Gigante Cushion, carefully place your toes on top the BOSU.

Note: I suggest you start with BOSU then attempt using the cushion. Wearing shoes helps versus being barefoot.

It is VERY challenging to lift one foot. Go easy. You might possibly crash onto the floor, so go easy. Good luck.

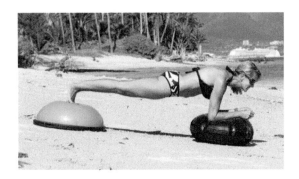 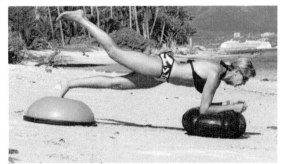

Exercise 3:
KNEE BALANCING ON STABILITY BALL WITH PROGRESSIONS

This is one of my favorites. Can you remember when you first stood up on a SUP board and your legs shook like wet noodles? Guys? For some reason guys have really weak adductor or inner thigh muscles. This is often the first thing many guys instantly tell me when I take them paddling for their first time. This exercise targets all the tiny finite muscles of the thigh up to the hips, as well as the deep pelvic floor muscles.

Again, you may "shake and bake," as I like to say, but in time your body will quiet down and all of the chaos you may feel at first will disappear. Your inner thighs are typically undertrained and need all the strength they can get. Don't give up because I know you want it! And I know you can do it!

You could also classify this exercise in the balance and brain training department, but for now it's really the core that will do the work.

SUGGESTED TRAINING EQUIPMENT
Large stability ball 55-65cm, chair, bench, or sturdy fixed object, 5-8 pound dumbbell or medicine ball, faith in yourself and courage

SUGGESTED REPS/SETS
1-3 sets, timed increments of 15 seconds, 30 seconds, 45 seconds, 1 minute

PROGRESSION VARIABLES
Soft ball to firm ball, hooked feet to unhooked feet, sturdy object to hands free, eyes open to eyes closed, no weights to added weight

If you've never tried this, please place the stability ball close to a sturdy object such as washing machine, bar top, or chair. If your ball is less full, it will be easier to get up. Now, carefully, one leg at a time, feet at hip width apart, place the shin part of your lower leg onto the ball and hook your toes behind you on the ball. You must bend slightly forward at the waist, eyes gazing forward not down. Breathe.

Note: *Don't ever come fully upright as this could cause strain to your lower back and cause you to fall.*

Now that you feel like a circus bear, your legs might be quivering and you might start to giggle. This is normal and I see it everyday. Keep up the good work.

PROGRESSION 1

Unhook your feet behind you. I call this removing the training wheels. Hips are still bent and you're leaning slightly forward.

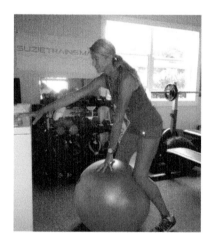 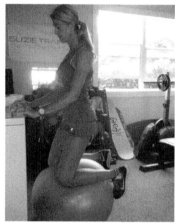 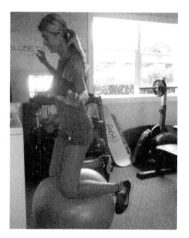

PROGRESSION 2

Slowly take one hand off whatever you are holding onto in front of you, then remove the other and see how long you can go without holding on. Time yourself in 15 second to two minute increments. It's a blast.

PROGRESSION 3

"Look no hands!"

Remove sturdy object but be sure to give yourself plenty of room in case you crash. It's not that bad if you do, but be careful.

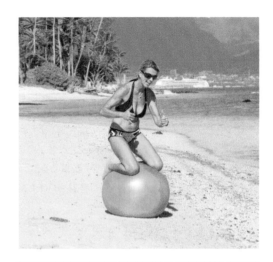

This is your goal.

PROGRESSION 4

From no hands we go to the ultimate proprioception stimulus by closing our eyes. You may want to start by holding onto something, which is totally fine. I highly suggest you hook your feet to help you if you need. Now close your eyes for just a few seconds then quickly open them. Did you crash? I hope not. What happened? Did you feel disoriented?

It's actually not too hard to do this, it's just that your brain literally has nothing to focus on but your movement.

PROGRESSION 5

Adding weights.

This is SUPER advanced. By now you can try out for Cirque du Soleil.

This changes everything. By adding weight to the exercise now we have a new force production going through certain points in our body directly to center of your core, hips, quads, glutes, inner thighs, and so forth.

If you take a weight such as an 8 pound medicine ball and move it from holding it close to your body to holding it away from your body, you will feel so many different muscles firing. The closer the ball to the center of effort, the easier the exercise will be. The second you move it away from your core, your world will change.

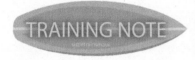
TRAINING NOTE

For example, as you reach for the nose of the board with your paddle your power is needed away from your core as well as in your core to grab the water for paddle purchase. When we stress our core with this exercise, we train our muscles to transfer power "outside" of our core while stabilizing on the ball. We use this type of movement when we have to stabilize our body on the board while paddling in tricky conditions while, at the same time, moving outside our core to get the board moving.

Setup: Place stability ball near a weight bench or chair in front of you. Give yourself some distance, maybe 2-3 feet, to mount up on the ball. Slowly reach for the 8 pound medicine ball—or 5 pound dumbbell if you like—and pick up with both hands. Hook your feet behind you and keep them there the entire exercise.

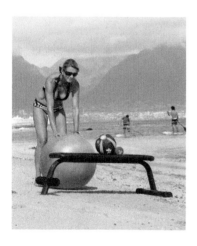
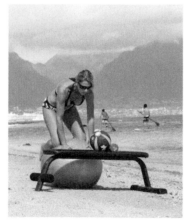
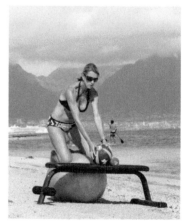

First, hold weight close to you, eyes forward. Next extend arms out in front of you and see how it feels and what happens. Be careful and focus. Good. As you become more comfortable increase the tempo of the above and maybe do this ten times. Be careful to add weight slowly. You can also hold medicine ball in one hand and move over the top of your head and repeat this ten times as well.

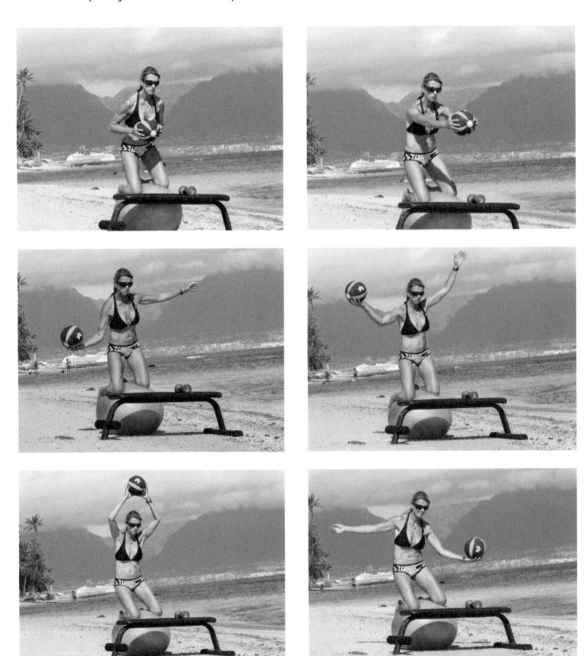

Return weight to bench. Good job! Now go hit the water and see if you can really find the power from your core.

Exercise 4:
ONE KNEE EXTREME CORE STABILIZING ON UNSTABLE PLATFORM / ALL PLANES OF MOTION

This exercise takes kneeling on the stability ball or cushion to the next level.

SUGGESTED TRAINING EQUIPMENT
Indo Board Gigante Cushion, BOSU 5-8 pound dumbbell or medicine ball.

SUGGESTED REPS/SETS
5-10 each leg, 1-2 sets

MOVEMENT TEMPO/SPEED
Controlled with 1-2 second holds

PROGRESSION VARIABLES
Firm inflation to less inflation, all planes of motion, eyes open to eyes closed, no weights to added weight

Place one knee on the Indo Board Logo of the Gigante Cushion (can also use BOSU) and do not let your foot touch behind you. Focus on something in front of you. Do not place your posture in full erect position, have a slight bend at your hips. Slowly extend the opposite leg in front, then to the side, then behind you. Repeat five times each leg.

Note: *The BOSU may be a better place to start, as the Gigante Cushion is very demanding. Remember—achieve good form first, then progress.*

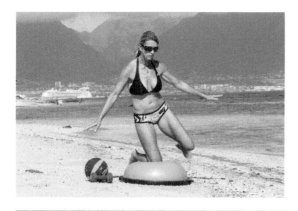
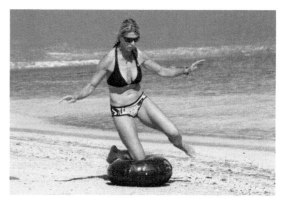

Some people will immediately notice their hips start to shake wildly. This is normal and will decrease in time as your brain begins to fire the correct stabilizing muscles around your femur. It's great for a giggle or two, and will dramatically calm itself as you practice. Keep at it.

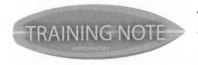

As your SUP skills begin to improve, I want you also to start thinking about the role your hips play in stand up paddling. Begin to pay attention to the dynamics of how your hips actually help thrust you slightly forward with each stroke. I teach this, I practice this, and I know it's true.

I mention this because it will start to happen for you too. Your hips are part of the driving force of power that help propel your board through the water from the moment your paddle enters the water to the time the blade exits.

For example, let's say you paddle into a choppy section. Your hips play a significant role in your total body strength, stabilizing you, driving and thrusting, as you navigate through. Is this making more sense now?

You need all of the hip muscles to be responsive and strong. We need to train the large and the tiny muscles to fire together and independently with each stroke.

This particular exercise will call upon the large and the finer muscles at the same time. We want to fatigue them all and train them hard so they do burn out. This is how build your "core" SUP endurance.

PROGRESSION 1

You still might be shaky but just go for it. Next while on one knee you'll attempt to move through all planes of motion. That means you'll bring your leg in front of you, to the side and then to rear. Like this:

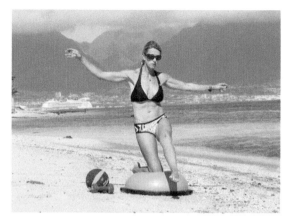 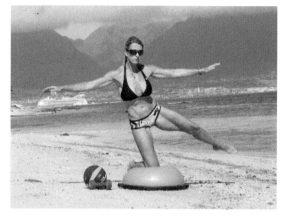

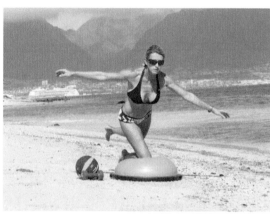 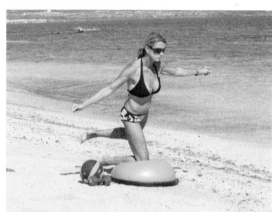

PROGRESSION 2

Pick up 5-8 pound medicine ball or dumbbell. While your leg is extended, move weight away from the center of your body at 12 o'clock, then to 2 o'clock, then back to 12 o'clock, and then to 10 o'clock. You can also move through all of the planes of motion while holding a medicine ball Repeat. Repeat five times, then switch knees.

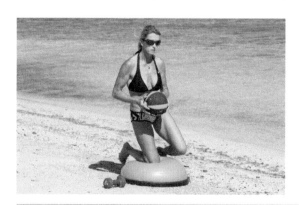 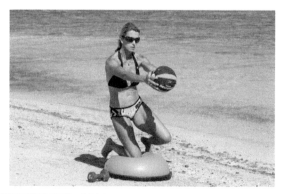

All Planes of Motion:

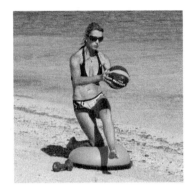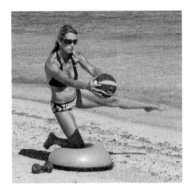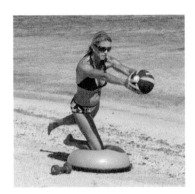

PROGRESSION 3

Without the weights, assume the first start position with one knee on the Gigante Cushion or BOSU while keeping in good postural alignment, hips slightly bent. Now simply close your eyes. Pretty crazy.

Exercise 5:
10 & 2'S: DYNAMIC CORE WITH UPPER BACK AND SHOULDER BENEFITS

This particular exercise really requires focus and concentration as it involves the upper back and shoulders to be your anchor. It's important to protect your lower back throughout each rep.

I love this one because people always say, "Wow I really feel that."

SUGGESTED TRAINING EQUIPMENT
Stability ball

SUGGESTED REPS/SETS
12-20 reps, 1-3 sets

PROGRESSION VARIABLES
Lower legs, increase range of motion from side to side

Begin by laying down on your mat. Place the stability ball between your legs and imagine yourself as a clock. Your head is 12 o'clock. To your left is 10 o'clock. To the right is 2 o'clock.

With the ball between both feet, lie back so your back is flat on the ground, your arms are out like a T, and your palms are pressed to the floor. Bend your knees slightly to assure no strain on your low back. This is your start position.

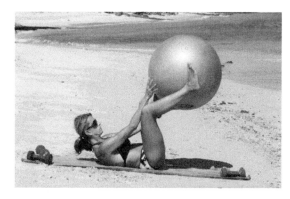

Next as you lower your legs slowly to 10 o'clock, or to the left; press your right

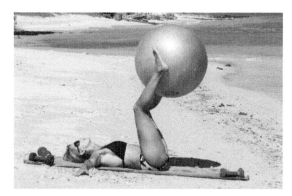

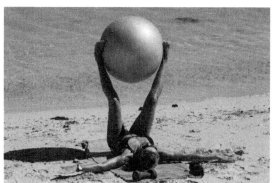

shoulder blade to the ground. It must stay securely and firmly there and not lift up. Only allow for your legs to get to 10 if you can keep that shoulder pressed. Engage your core muscles, gently squeeze the ball with feet to add more juice if you can, and bring the ball back to center or 12 o'clock. Breathe. Wow, right?!

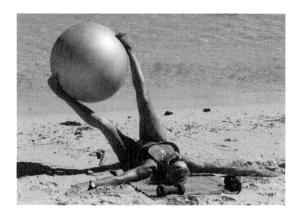

Then, while pressing left shoulder blade to ground, allow for your legs to fall toward the right, or 2 o'clock, and use all your might in your core to bring ball back to start, or 12 o'clock.

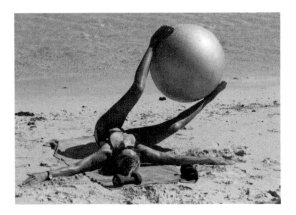

PROGRESSION 1

Slightly lower legs towards ground, avoid arching of lower back.

Exercise 6:
DYNAMIC CORE PADDLING OBLIQUE STABILIZATION TO POWER

I saved the best for last. In the above core exercises I offered you variety, from basic to advanced. Now you should have the core concept down and are ready to go up one more level.

This exercise requires one to understand how to engage the core muscles before starting and throughout the entire set of the exercise. *You* become the stabilizing factor as you perform these exercises. Also, I'd like you to pay attention to the fact that, during the entire set, the tubing you use or TRX Rip Trainer cord will always be taut and under tension. This can be called "time under tension." If you "let go" of this concept or your core, your stroke will not be as powerful as it can be.

SUGGESTED TRAINING EQUIPMENT

TRX Rip Trainer (heavy cord is best), 4-8 pound dumbbell, Indo Board Gigante Cushion and/or BOSU, Indo Board Pro Kicktail Board or Rocker Board (less advanced)

SUGGESTED REPS/SETS

1-3 sets, timed increments of 15 seconds, 30 seconds, 45 seconds, 1 minute+, or you can count 20, 25 strokes, and so forth

PROGRESSION VARIABLES

Ground to unstable platform, medium gauge cord to heavy, lighter medicine ball to heavier, or 4-8 pound dumbbell, low cadence to high cadence

Secure the TRX Rip Trainer cord to a sturdy, secure object. Make sure you have enough room for proper execution and full strokes.

Start with your feet solidly planted on the ground at about shoulder width, pointed straight. Stand with good posture, knees slightly bent, eyes forward. Hold the TRX bar with the right hand on top, left hand toward the bottom just below the top of your shoulder. Begin to engage your core by drawing in your abs and holding—but keep breathing.

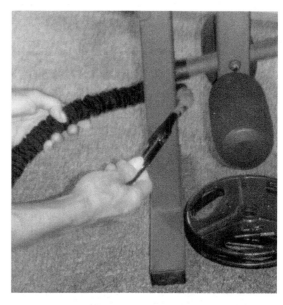

(Remember, safety loop!) Do not keep a death grip on the bar but start far enough away from post with enough tension that will require you to stabilize the bar and your body. As you reach forward toward the left side of your body, like you reach forward with your paddle toward the nose of your board, allow the cord to loosen slightly. Imagine

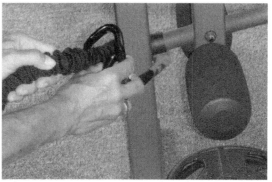

your paddle blade entering the water and at that second, BOOM, turn on your left deep obliques. Smoothly pull the TRX Rip Trainer cord back towards your feet in a controlled, straight line but DO NOT pull too far past your feet. Complete the stroke with obliques still turned on.

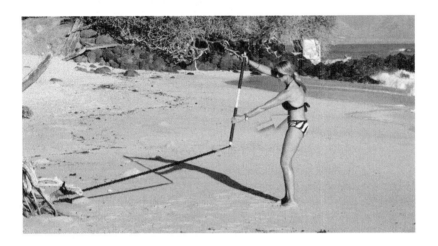

The ability to turn on one side of your body's obliques may take some concentration and time. Keep at it. The "feeling" I'm talking about will soon become natural.

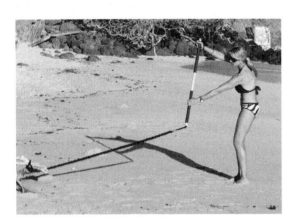 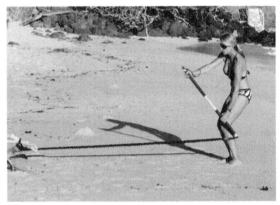

Repeat and continue. Fool around with tension and cadence. Always stay in control and keep breathing. You can time yourself or you can give yourself goals in increments of, for example, 25+ strokes on each side, maybe two sets on each side. Or two sets of one minute each side. Or, say, in a two minute period, start out slowly, increase cadence and then turn it down again. Repeat as you would if you were interval training.

PROGRESSION 1

Change the platform you are standing on or use a heavier gauge tubing/cord. Now we go from stable to unstable, which allows you simulate changing water conditions.

Stand on BOSU or other unstable platform. INDO Board Kicktail on top of Gigante Cushion is very challenging. Mess around with different inflation levels, as that can totally change the behavior of your TRX training.

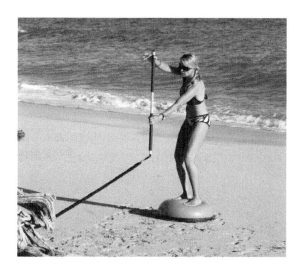
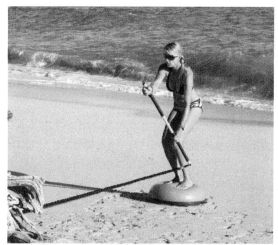
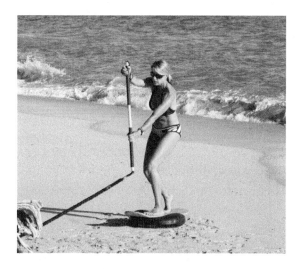
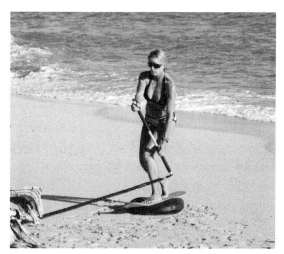

PROGRESSION 2

Replace the TRX Rip Trainer with a 4-8 pound medicine ball or dumbbell

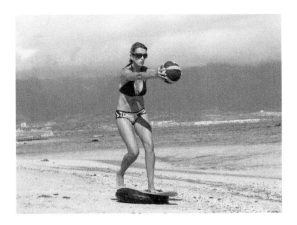 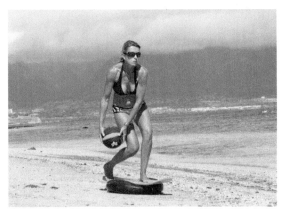

This is fun to try as well. As you reach with each stroke, remember to engage your obliques and try not to put too much stress on your arms. Reduce amount of weight if necessary to maintain good form. Stroke and train on.

Keep up the good work and the more you can really get this down, the more energy you'll have to spare from the rest of your body. By having the strongest possible core you'll cruise the finish with reserves to spare.

I hope you've enjoyed just a small sample of my selected core exercises with stand up paddling in mind. There are many more that I perform with my clients in my studio or on the beach.

The key is to be able to perform all of these in a smooth, controlled manner without any deviations in your posture or form. Go easy and don't push too hard too soon.

If you paddle with a weak core your performance will suffer. It's probably pretty hard to over-train your core, but it's not entirely impossible. Once your core is solid then we'll be able to move on the next step in getting a stronger body for stand up paddling, and that is balance.

Next up, I'll show you some of favorite ab exercises.

AB EXERCISES: ABSOLUTELY WE MUST TRAIN THE ABS

What kind of trainer would I be if we did not include the abs? But first we need clarify that the abs are an accessory of the total core set of muscles and will be trained separately.

When you read Chapter 9 you will learn how to develop your own training program and you'll be able to plug in these exercises. Just to let you know now, you'll perform your ab exercises last because your abs support you all throughout your workout.

Exercise 1:
CHEST LIFTS - THE BEST EXERCISE TO TARGET LOWER & UPPER ABS

I "AB-solutely" love these. Sorry, I could not resist. If you love your ab exercises your abs will love you back and help you power your core to the finish. So start loving them. These are the best ab exercise to get to the lower abs at the same time and they don't hurt your neck. Huge bonus.

The chest lifts are called this because it's actually your chest lifting towards the ceiling to contract and activate your upper and lower abs.

SUGGESTED TRAINING EQUIPMENT
Self

SUGGESTED REPS/SETS
25-125 reps, 1-3 sets

PROGRESSION VARIABLES
Leg upright to lower leg position to max out lower abs

Extend either leg and lift slightly off floor. If you experience any lower back discomfort, raise the extended leg higher. Bend the knee of the opposite leg. Hold hands behind your head and DO NOT lock fingers. Gently support head in nape of neck with fingertips.

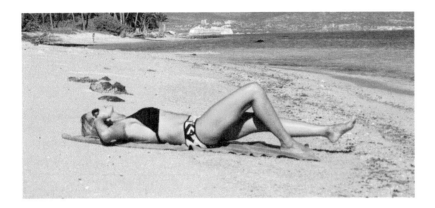

Imagine a pulley on your chest lifting you to the ceiling. Make sure you are looking above your eyebrow to prevent elbows from falling forward.

Lift chest / shoulders off floor and enforce your abs to contract. As you lift, hold that contraction for a count of two and breathe out. DO NOT allow your shoulders to come back to floor, but keep the abs taught at all times.

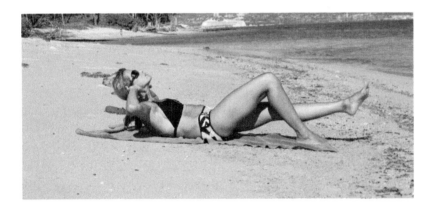

If you notice your elbows winging forward, look up and flatten them out, otherwise your neck will become sore and the exercise will have little affect.

Please be sure to do your best and get through the burn. Press your fingers into nape of your neck to help support your head.

The shaking is normal. It will get less and less! Keep at it and always add ten more at the finish!

Exercise 2:
MEDICINE BALL LIFTS

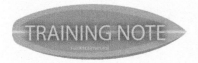 *If you are just beginning a training program I highly recommend you start with little to no weight so you don't stress your lower back.*

I like to get the most bang for my rep and this is it. You will get stronger abs with each stroke so get to it. This ab exercise is amazing.

SUGGESTED TRAINING EQUIPMENT
Medicine ball or dumbbell, 4-10 pounds

SUGGESTED REPS/SETS
1-3 sets center abs and 10 – 15 on obliques right and left

PROGRESSION VARIABLES
Hold for 2 seconds, increase weight

Sit on mat with medicine ball in front of you, knees in front of you and slightly bent. Roll down toward mat, keeping the back flat with a slight bend in the elbow. Relax your neck.

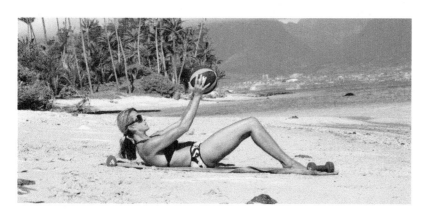

Keep feet glued to ground as you lift the medicine ball toward the ceiling. The range of motion is small on your first rep. Don't let your feet come up off the ground. Return back to the mat—but don't let your shoulders touch the mat—and continue. Breathe out with each rep up.

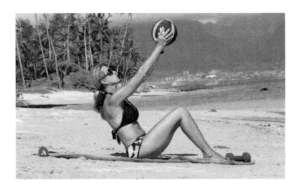

Next, obliques: Simply sit on your right hip bone, bend knees, and, this time use your obliques to lift you. You should be locked in the pocket of the obliques with each rep. What I do is keep them turned on throughout the entire set.

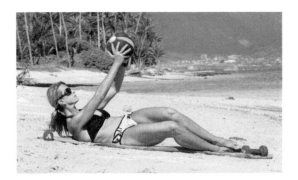 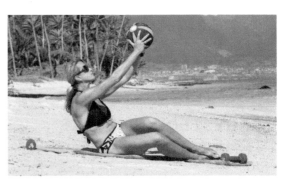

Exercise 3:
BOSU AB BLAST

This one is a killer, but you will want to learn to love it. If you want to get the obliques to really fire and be strong for a strong stroke, this is a GREAT exercise.

SUGGESTED TRAINING EQUIPMENT
BOSU

SUGGESTED REPS/SETS
20-25 reps, 1-3 sets, each side: center and obliques

PROGRESSION VARIABLES
Hold for 2 seconds

Forward Position for Center Abs: Sit on top of the BOSU just below the circle. Place your hands behind you on the BOSU and lean back slightly with knees bent. You'll feel your abs contract and pooch out. This is good.

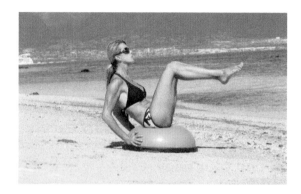 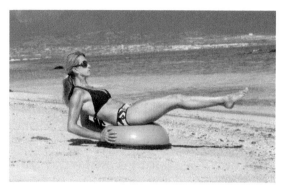

Bring your knees towards you and contract your abs. Hold for 1-2 seconds, return to start with knees bent, repeat.

Side, Oblique Position Left or Right: Sit with your right or left hip bone on top circle with one hand behind you and the other to the side; both on the BOSU. Like the exercise above, knees are bent and now you'll feel the obliques firing!

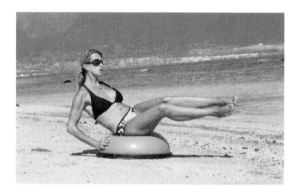 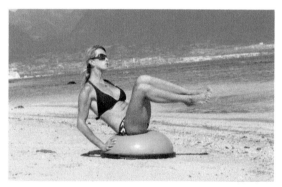

This will be awkward at first, but do your best. Bring your knees towards you and contract your abs. Hold for 1-2 seconds, return to start with knees bent, repeat.

As I close this chapter I imagine that now you're making a much better connection to your abs and core muscles. The connection to your paddling performance is "AB-solutely" huge and the training will pay off with every stroke!

Now get ready for lots of fun balance work to work on your leg and reaction training so you can paddle and stay standing in any and all conditions!

CHAPTER 3
How to Improve Your Balance:
Brain Training to be One with the Board

- Why you need excellent balance to be a stronger SUP paddler.
- The brain's connection to your paddle and to your SUP board: Reaction and speed training.
- Learning to let go and trust the board and your body.
- Balance exercises that will launch your balance from horrible to amazing.

Ever notice how some people appear to have Spiderman-like reflexes and are able to stay on their SUP boards in the most insane conditions? How do you do when you attempt to surf up and over a small wave like in this photo of me on Maui?

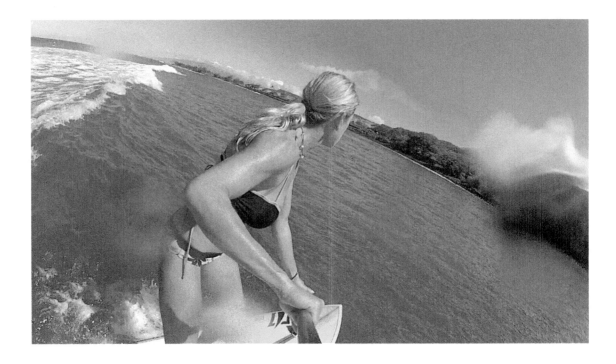

Think back when you first started getting into stand up paddling. Maybe you fell a lot at first? Or were you one of those who just got up and paddled off into the sunset?

After all these years of teaching people to paddle, one thing that really stands out is the continuous need to balance train. This also includes me. Excellent balance is critical if you want to go to the next level of stand up paddling. This also applies to flat water specialists.

WHY YOU NEED EXCELLENT BALANCE TO BE A STRONGER SUP PADDLER:

I've written tons of articles and produced videos on how to improve your balance for stand up paddling and here is where I really break it down.

Time and time again my clients and I notice a **HUGE** difference when we put time into balance training on land. Right away they notice how they could transfer that extra special skill from their body to stay upright in small surf, big surf, or to catch more bumps and glides.

When you spend time on balance training, continuously improving your balance, your confidence and SUP skills will soar. You will be completely amazed at how you can save yourself from falling, stay upright while paddling through side chop, or stay on your board while rounding a buoy through a crowd during a difficult race turn.

Most people rely on their large muscles such as the hip, the knee, and the ankle to push themselves through a bottom turn, to catch a glide on a downwinder, or to take off during a sprint race. However, if you can call upon all of your tiny finer muscles to fire first and then signal the larger muscles to jump in, your performance will increase ten-fold.

For instance, flat water paddlers also need good balance to keep all of the teeny tiny muscles we train around the major joints, such as the hip, knees, and ankles from becoming fatigued.

THE BRAIN CONNECTION TO YOUR PADDLE AND TO YOUR SUP BOARD:REACTION AND SPEED TRAINING

Think you're quick? I know I'm quick. My reflexes were tested at an early age by my father in preparation for dirt bike racing. Later I honed those skills and put them to test windsurfing. Then along came SUP and after breaking both ankles and one leg in 2009 I was deflated and had to relearn all those years of being "fast." I had to learn to walk again! When I first started to SUP I was slooooooow.

Having quick reflexes goes hand in hand with having good balance. You can improve the way your brain responds to changing water conditions, like chop to small or big waves.

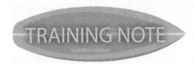

Reflexes: *An action that is performed as a response to a stimulus and without conscious thought. Some people are quick and cat-like, others, well, turtle-like. You need reflexes in life and you need them for SUP.*

Think of this for a moment: If you're racing and rounding a buoy are you anticipating the next actions of the people around you? What is your reaction? Are you ready to block or pass? Or, to digress to my dirt bike days, the gate drops into the first turn and you're heading into a banking berm on the dirt bike track. To avoid locking handlebars in such a critical moment you need to be able to react fast and keep your limbs tight to the bike.

Here's another common one for SUP: You have the right of way and you're about to have a water disaster with another paddler, or worse, a surfer. Is your brain going to connect fast enough to the rest of your body to actually do what you need to do to get out of the way, rather than just *thinking* about what you need to do?

Another term we'll use here is proprioception training. In technical terms it means "The cumulative sensory input to the central nervous system from all mechanorecptors that sense body position and limb movement" (NASM National Academy Sports Medicine Personal Fitness Training 3rd Edition). What that simply means is that the better your brain is trained with proprioception work or by working on your balance, the better you'll perform on the water.

The reason I share all of this with you is because as you learn the exercises I present, the progression variables are a little crazy. However, the better you become at these exercises and the more you know "why" they are important, the better paddler you'll become.

LEARNING TO LET GO AND TRUST THE BOARD AND YOUR BODY

Before we go into these particular balance exercises, I'd like you to picture yourself in your mind conquering each one in time. (Common sense rules, though!) If you feel frustrated at first, go slow and try to be patient. It takes time for your brain to register new information. With each attempt it learns and remembers more.

People trust me that I will set them up for success. That is my desire for you. Now you need to let go and try and new things in order to be a stronger stand up paddler.

I've noticed some people I train like to be in control of everything in their environment. This can be a fatal outlook and is all but impossible in SUP. Variables that you have no control over are constantly changing—from wind direction to swell, and even positions of other paddlers. You *must* learn how to quickly react to variables outside your control.

Sometimes I purposely and sneakily introduce new balance challenges and brain tests to these kinds of people. I never set anyone up to fail; I simply create an environment and safe space to try new things and get people out of their comfort zone—all within reason and common sense to their ability level.

At first, they look at me as if I have three heads. It's amazing how they surprise themselves when they actually perform well. I have faith in you and you should too. When I'm scared on the top of a wave that is bigger than what I first thought I say to myself, "Go! This is what you do!"

I let go and trust the board.

BALANCE EXERCISES

These are my favorite super cool balance exercises that will help you launch your balance from horrible to amazing.

These exercises are crazy fun and challenging and, like everything we do, you must master good form for each exercise before you progress to the more difficult exercises or to the more difficult progressions within each exercise. Just as you do with the core exercises, add 2-3 of these balance exercises to your workout each day and keep mixing them up.

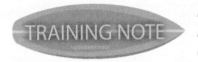

Be sure to go to my You Tube Channel: http://bit.ly/1VxpbWD and you can see some of these exercises there too.

Just as in Chapter 2, the progressions for each exercise start with the least challenging and move to the maximum level of difficulty for each exercise.

Some people prefer to be barefoot while doing balance exercises. I personally do the exercises both while barefoot and while wearing shoes. For example, I like to feel the Indo Board, so I prefer to do those exercises without shoes. Whatever you're most comfortable doing is great. Be sure to give yourself enough space in case you crash and, if possible, make sure the ground underneath you is not just hard cement. I use Indo Board's special training carpet for added grip and for softer landings.

Exercise 1:
BALANCE BASICS IN ALL PLANES OF MOTION

As a trainer and paddler, I want to introduce a new concept that will help keep your brain and stand up paddling skills extra sharp in *all dimensions*. Now, it's critical you don't rush through these exercises, as you'll see in the grand finale of these balance challenges. The last one will take your breath away...or your paddle.

What I mean by this is that we live and paddle in one dimension. We walk forward, we swim forward, we surf forward, and we all can say we paddle forward. Sure, we turn, we cut back, and I have seen some paddle backwards to goof off, but we usually train and paddle in one dimension.

Now I have experienced, not on purpose, the act of sliding sideways on a big downwind glide. It's almost like drifting in a racecar or doing, what we call in the rally world, a 4-point drift. Have you ever felt your board skid sideways? What did you do? How did you react? Did you fight it or did you think it was way cool and go with it?

I want to tune you in to something that I do here in the studio or at the beach with some of my SUP folks without them even realizing it. I'm training their brain to paddle and be in all dimensions at every moment. It's not voodoo or island magic; it's called training in different "dimensions" or "planes" of motion. I have my clients do this with force, no force, with weights or without weights. (We will go deeper into this when we talk about bracing.)

For example we paddle forward on the right or left side of board in the **sagittal** plane, then we look and twist with our lower body to catch a wave or turn around a buoy in the **transverse** plane or lower superior of body. Sometimes when you're doing a cut back, you're paddling in all planes at once. As your board is sliding or floating across the lip of the wave you are now in the coronal or **frontal** plane.

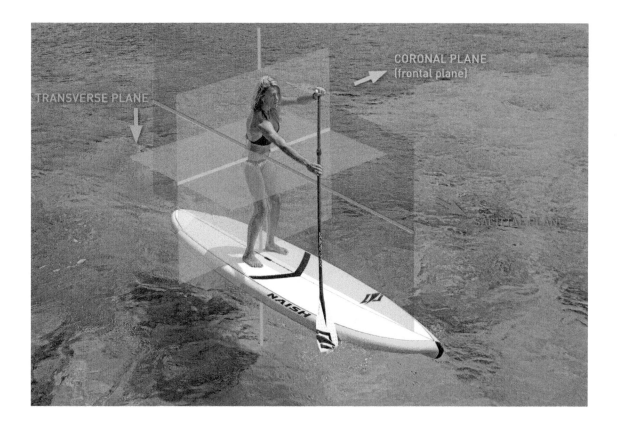

THREE PRIMARY ANATOMICAL PLANES OF MOTION

Sagittal plane: divides body into right and left sides – We paddle on the left or right side of the board. Bracing with paddle lands us here.

Frontal plane: divides body into front/back – We respond, react and shift our weight as needed to recover, catch a bump or catch a wave here.

Transverse plane: divides body into top and bottom – We compress, uncoil, recoil, thrust, twist body in opposite direction for cut back, floater or to step turn into a wave.

Now you have a visual of training in all dimensions! When you challenge the muscles and stimulate joint actions that are not in their normal, known pattern or path, you'll be taking your body into new training dimensions of planes of motion. This truly is the ultimate for any level of stand up paddler.

SUGGESTED TRAINING EQUIPMENT
Half foam roller, INDO Board 12" disc and/or 24" Gigante Cushion Pro Kicktail (most difficult) or any other Indo Board Platform will do, (1) BOSU

SUGGESTED REPS/SETS
10-12 each leg, 1-2 sets

MOVEMENT TEMPO/SPEED
Controlled with 1-5 second holds

PROGRESSION VARIABLES
2- 1 leg, floor to 12 inch half foam roller, to Indo Boards + 12" and/or 24" Gigante Cushion, all planes of motion, eyes open to closed

PROGRESSION 1

Stand with two feet on the ground, then simply lift one leg and point your toes in front of you, then to the side, and then behind you. Congratulations, you've just entered into all planes of motion balance training. Repeat suggested reps/sets with other leg. You can also hold your leg in any plane of motion up to 5 seconds to increase the intensity and challenge. Squeeze your butt on the back side of the frontal plane or behind you for extra glute strength.

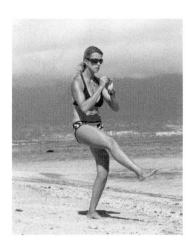
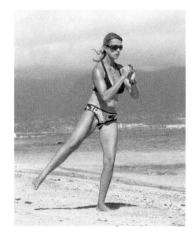
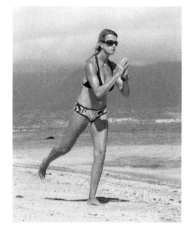

PROGRESSION 2

Repeat the above first progression, this time with your eyes closed. I'm serious. This is training the brain to the max. Be careful and use precaution. The hardest part will be when you open your eyes and you have to reset and focus on something. Crazy fun! If you're nervous, maybe hold on to a sturdy object at first.

PROGRESSION 3

Now we simply step up, literally, to the 12 inch half foam dense roller to add some medial and lateral movement (left to right, inside to out) to the balance challenge. Start by simply balancing on your right leg with a slightly bent knee. Add your new trick, moving through all planes of motion. Repeat on the left leg. Then, just like you did in Progression 2, close your eyes! Cool, huh? Master this before moving on up to the BOSU.

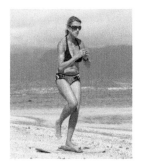
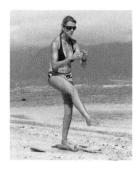
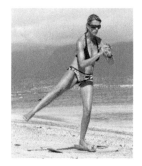
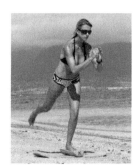

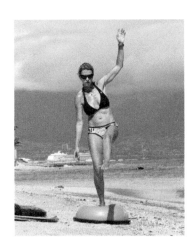 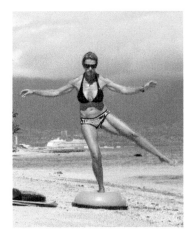 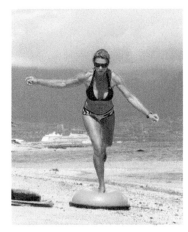

PROGRESSION 4

Take the half foam roller and place on the ground horizontally. Step up with two feet with feet about 4 inches apart but not hanging over the edge. Keep both knees bent. Don't look down—look forward, hands off your body. Relax and breathe. Once you've settled in, keep your upper body as quiet as possible.

Put your arms in front of you and attempt a few little squats.

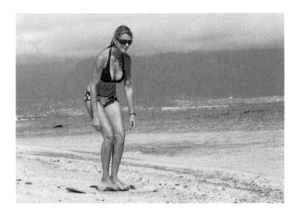

If your arms start to flail or move backwards or forwards in big large circles, I call that "rolling down the windows." You want to (and will!) get to the point where this doesn't happen.

Now do this with eyes closed. . . seriously there's no need to get out mouth guard. Trust yourself. Ready to rock and roll? It just keeps getting better!

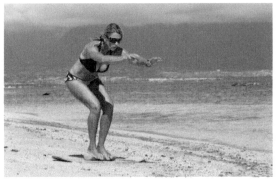

PROGRESSION 5

Grab your 12 inch or 24 inch Indo Board Gigante Cushion and Indo Board of choice (Pro Kicktail is the most challenging) and center board on top of cushion **nubby side up**. Now, confidently, as in Progression 1, place one foot in center, bend knee and begin your all planes of motion challenge here. It's great fun! After five or so, switch to opposite leg.

Then, of course, close your eyes for a few seconds.

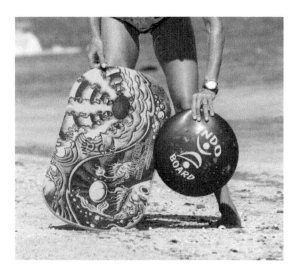
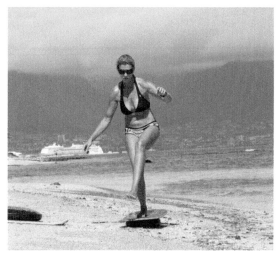
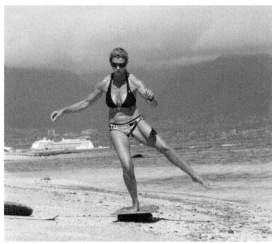
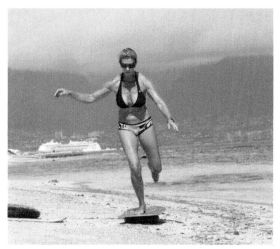

Congrats on your first test of balance. Now you have excellent balance. Say it out loud, do it, be one with it.

Exercise 2:
SINGLE LEG TOE REACH
refer to http://bit.ly/1XidgO9

The level of mental focus of this exercise is incredibly high. You will burn extra calories for sure. This exercise could also fit into the leg strength section, Chapter 5, but for now I want this to be all about balance. The strength you'll gain is an added bonus!

You may feel your foot catch on fire. That's a sign that you need to release your toes from grabbing the ground or board! Relax, breathe, and concentrate on every muscle.

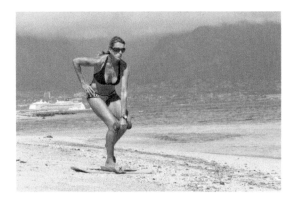

SUGGESTED TRAINING EQUIPMENT
Dumbbells 5-10 pounds, half foam roller, Indo Board 24" Gigante Cushion deflated 30%, Indo Board Pro Kicktail (most difficult) or any other Indo Board Platform will do. I also recommend a full-length mirror so you can see your postural alignment.

SUGGESTED REPS/SETS
10-12 each leg, 1-2 sets

MOVEMENT TEMPO/SPEED
Controlled with 1-5s hold at bottom before you rise back to the start position

PROGRESSION VARIABLES
Floor to half foam roller, to Indo Board Gigante Cushion, no weight to dumbbell, 1-5 seconds

PROGRESSION 1

Begin on the floor, balanced on your right leg with your knee slightly bent (15-20 degrees). Keep your right hand on your right hip. Draw your abdomen inward toward your belly button for spinal stabilization. Without allowing further knee movement, bend over at the hip, trying to touch down with the opposite hand. Look in the mirror and make sure your kneecap is tracking over your second toe.

Push through the heel back to start position, fully upright.

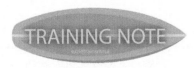

When I do any form of these, I will sometimes place a surf key in front of my foot to have a focus point or a speck in the carpet or floor. It gives my brain something to grab.

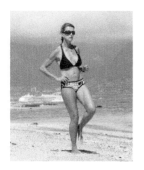 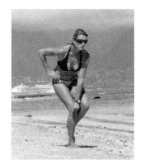 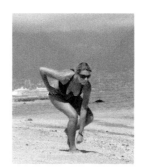 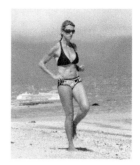

PROGRESSION 2

Start same way as in Progression 1, but now let's add some weight. Pick up a dumbbell with the left hand and keep near your hip with elbow bent. By adding a weight you will feel the intensity rise, which is all the more reason not to grab the floor with your toes. Start easy. If you increase the weight this also counts for leg strengthening. By adding weight we add a load to all of the muscles during this balance challenge, which causes the small muscles to fatigue quickly. I would not add more than ten pounds here.

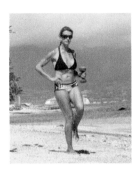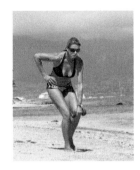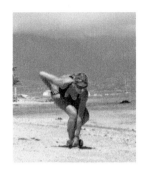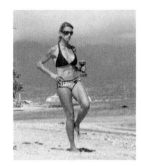

PROGRESSION 3

Moving up to the dense half foam roller, we add a medial to lateral challenge, or left to right, inside to outside of knee line. This takes time, and it might be challenging to keep your knee tracking straight, but do your best. Start with no weight, then pick up a dumbbell.

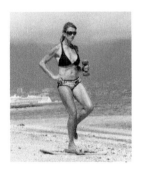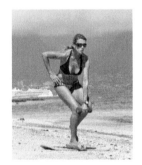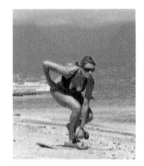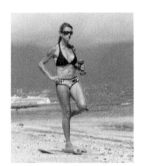

PROGRESSION 4

Begin with Gigante Cushion, nubby side up, and place and position your choice of Indo Board in center. Here, the Gigante Flo cushion is inflated at about 30%. Place your right foot on the center of the Indo Board, knee slightly bent, left foot nearby to spot. Do this with good posture, no weights. Slowly bend at right hip, and reach with left hand to top of foot without looking down at it. Hold for 2-5 seconds to increase challenge and intensity and add a dumbbell.

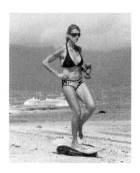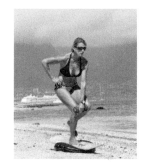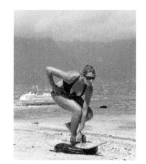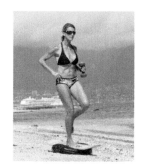

Exercise 3:
CATCH A WAVE ON THE INDO BOARD

After completing the challenging exercises above, you aren't ready for JAWS just yet. You might be reading this in Kansas and dreaming about waves. It doesn't matter if you're a flat water racer, just love to explore, or you might actually want paddle into JAWS someday, one can't get enough balance training.

For some this will be back to the basics because Indo Board has led the way for years in land surfing. It's still important to keep your skills sharp, no matter how much experience you have.

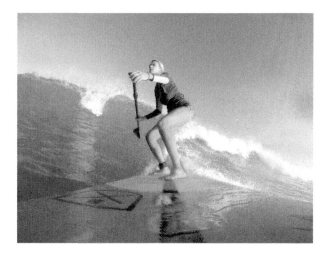

I'm going to give you some new cues to learn, so that everyone, even the most seasoned paddlers, will have something new to try. As always, safety comes first, so use your head and take precaution so you don't fall on it.

SUGGESTED TRAINING EQUIPMENT

INDO Board small roller (5" in diameter) and/or larger roller (8.5 inches in diameter) carpet, sand, foam padding or rubber mat will do.

SUGGESTED SURFING SESSIONS

Timed, controlled, safe. You can time yourself for 30 seconds to 5 minutes as long as you are: A. Not hungover B. Keep both eyes open and forward C. Progress safely D. All the above

PROGRESSION VARIABLES

Holding onto stationary object, then without. Surfing stance from 1-3 positions. There are some great videos to watch with techniques ranging from basic to advanced. Check out *IndoBoard.com*

PROGRESSION 1

I like to start people on the smaller roller, holding on to a stationary bike with me spotting them. Just like stand up paddling, at first, if you need, you can look down to get your footing, but it's important that you then train your eyes forward. Place the board atop the roller with the right edge touching the ground. Place your right foot on the board as you are holding onto a sturdy object and then place the left foot, equal distance apart. Slightly bend your knees and keep your eyes forward.

The board will move left to right. Gently apply pressure so you can get the feel of how the roller and board respond to your shift in weight. Go easy. To dismount safely, gently tap the Indo Board with your right foot down to the ground and always step off behind the roller. Never dismount off the Indo Board and roller in front of the roller. Practice dismounting safely a few times so you get used to getting on and off before we go to Progression 2.

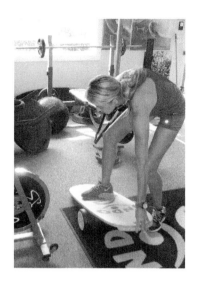
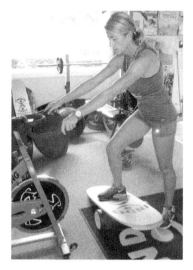
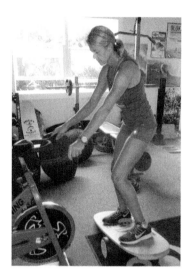

PROGRESSION 2

Okay surfers, now let's change directions. It doesn't matter if you don't know if you're goofy foot (right foot) forward or regular (left foot) foot forward. Step up to the standard position, knees bent, hanging onto your sturdy object and slowly turn your feet to left or right. (You may look down to position your feet.) Now look in the direction you are surfing. Good job.

Move back to standard position then turn to the other direction. Go easy, keep knees bent and eyes looking forward.

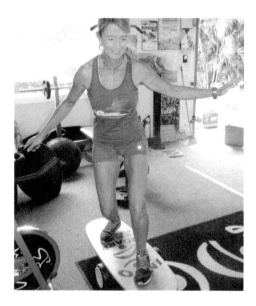
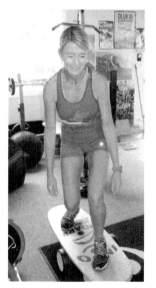

PROGRESSION 3

Once you've mastered the above and can comfortably do it without holding onto anything, you can now have your first solo balance surf session. Next let's have you turn your feet to the left. Hold that position for 10-15 seconds, come back to standard position and then try it in the other direction.

Do you feel more balanced goofy or regular? If you are getting into SUP surfing, I encourage you to learn both directions because it is nice to show up to a surf break knowing how to paddle surf front side and back side. I love doing this at the beach. Here the shot is on hard-pack sand and downhill.

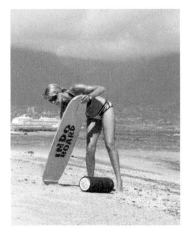 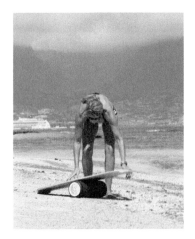 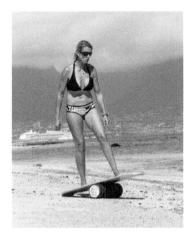

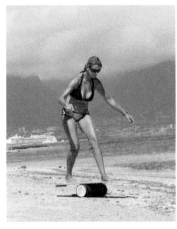 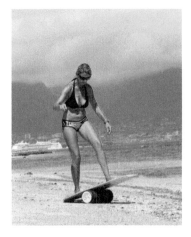 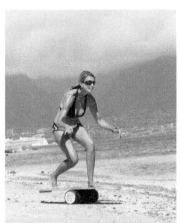

Exercise 4:
ULTIMATE REFLEX CHALLENGE

Now we get to increase your paddle reach to water speed. As you prepare for the final exercise in this chapter, we need to test and build your response speed. Your environment where you're practicing this exercise is controlled but the water is not. You can't read the water's or competitor's mind, so you need to be ready to respond.

I have a short video on my Suzie Cooney YouTube Channel "All-in-One Workout: How to Improve Balance, Core and Reflexes." Check it out here: *http://bit.ly/1OazVpl*

The idea here is to be light on your feet and light on your board. Get your hands and feet moving and get into a rhythm.

SUGGESTED TRAINING EQUIPMENT

Half foam 12 inch roller, small hard rubber ball (air filled), BOSU, Indo Board 24" Gigante Cushion, Indo Board Pro Kicktail (most difficult) or any other Indo Board Platform will do, Indo Board small (5" in diameter) and/or larger roller (8.5 inches in diameter), stability ball

SUGGESTED REPS/SETS

5-25+ reps

PROGRESSION VARIABLES

Endless! 2 to 1 leg, ground to unstable platform, right hand to left hand

PROGRESSION 1

The BOSU is your target. Place BOSU dome side up and find a spot just below the center circle. This is where you will focus your gaze. If you want, at first, you can place a small sticker in that spot, but in time you will want to remove it.

Stand on the balls of your feet with your two feet about 3 feet away from the Bosu. Throw the ball firmly against that sticker and try to catch it when it bounces back.

How's your toss? You'll need to be as consistent as possible with your throw. Get up on the balls of your feet and move and around.

Now switch to the opposite hand and throw. How did that go? Keep trying

PROGRESSION 2

Next grab the Indo Board Gigante Cushion with the Pro Kicktail and step up with two feet. Keep your knees bent at all times. Focus and breathe! Crazy! Now do the left, and then both.

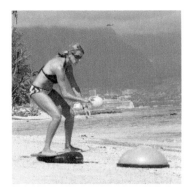 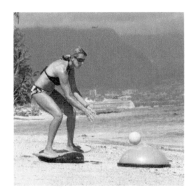 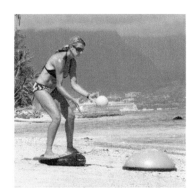

PROGRESSION 3

THIS is going to be fun! Now that your core is getting stronger, let's get on our knees on the stability ball and rock the house. You may ask a friend to catch the ball for you as getting on and off the stability ball will get tiring. Just don't miss. On this exercise it's okay to grab the stability ball with your feet. Keep your hips bent and go for it. Have fun because each throw is different and there is no sweet spot.

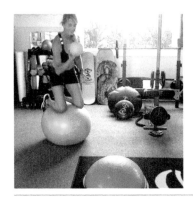 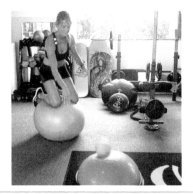 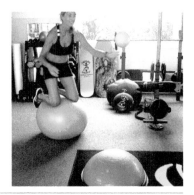

PROGRESSION 4

Select either the 12 inch or 24 inch Indo Board Cushion and your board of choice. There are three positions to work on:
1. 2 feet on board
2. 1 foot on board
3. surf stance

Prepare as you did from Progression 1 and give it your best shot.

Exercise 5:
BALANCE FOR BRACING: LET'S PADDLE

Do you know how to brace yourself with your paddle before you fall? Can you instinctively plant your paddle without looking and confidently know it will be exactly where you need it, without falling off your board? Are you having trouble with quick turns into a wave or around a buoy?

When you specifically balance train to brace with your paddle, you'll be storing unique imprints of body reactions from your brain to the paddle to the water. You'll be able to recall that imprint of information your brain has learned at any moment exactly when you need it.

For those learning to SUP surf: Have you practiced, time and time again, hopping up over that small or medium sized wave or beach break attempting to get out, only to find yourself quickly stepping (or running or falling) off the nose or back of board? These exercises will help you get up and over that small or medium size chop or wave and help you brace with your paddle to prevent a fall.

After working on these exercises, the next time you're pushing the paddle off the lip, or free falling maybe a bit sideways down the face of a big wave, or air dropping down the "back" side of a small wave your brain will instinctively put your paddle in the right place because you have trained it.

You can see a lot of these moves and more on video: click here: *http://bit.ly/1L6z7yK*

Safety Note: *Perform these exercises on the grass or sand, not cement or hard surface, to protect yourself if you fall and to protect your paddle. Also, you may not want to use your best paddle in case you land too hard. A broom or flexible stick works well too! You can choose to be barefoot or in shoes. You should not do this exercise if you have any ankle or knee injuries.*

SUGGESTED TRAINING EQUIPMENT

BOSU, SUP Board preferably 10 ft or under (no fins) Indo Board small (5" in in diameter) and/or larger roller (8.5 inches in diameter) Indo Board Kicktail Pro or any Indo Board, Indo Board Gigante Cushion, an older, junk paddle—broom works great—carpet, foam grass, sand, padding or rubber mat will do

PROGRESSION VARIABLES

Normal paddle stance to surf stance, floor to Indo Board, Gigante Cushion to SUP board, 50% inflation of Gigante Cushion to maximum inflation. Indo Board Roller plus Indo Board Pro Board to actual SUP board on top of fully maxed out Gigante Cushion

PROGRESSION 1

First position is two feet on the BOSU at about shoulder width apart with your paddle in hand in a horizontal position. Bend your knees to at least a 90 degree angle and reach out with your paddle in a fast, quick reach to the right Place your feet at about 2 or 3 o'clock (if you're facing 12 o'clock) and hold the paddle with the flat side of blade to the ground. Now put just a touch of your body weight in to it.

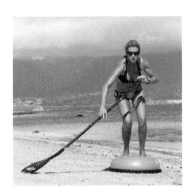 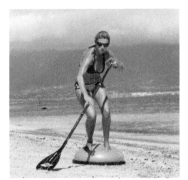 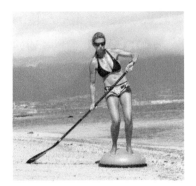

IMPORTANT NOTE: *Keep your eyes directed forward—not following your paddle.*

Repeat to the left side, between 9 and 11 o'clock, and lean into that. You can switch back and forth left to right, or do five in each position.

Next, still in same stance, pretend you are starting to fall backwards. Reach behind your hips and shoulder with your paddle. On the clock, this would be at about 4 o'clock to the right and opposite side, near 8 o'clock. Same important note applies: Keep your eyes focused forward; don't be tempted to look behind you. If you do in real life, you are guaranteed to fall.

Cool! You're officially bracing in all planes of motion.

PROGRESSION 2

Inflate Indo Board Gigante Cushion to about 80%. With the nubby side up, place the board of your choice on top. Now we start to feel a 4 way directional challenge. This is super fun. Simply repeat everything you learned above in Progression 1 and then add preferred surf stance.

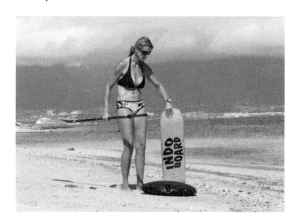
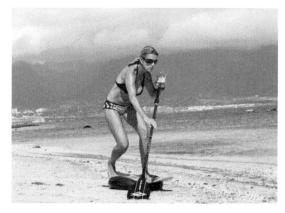
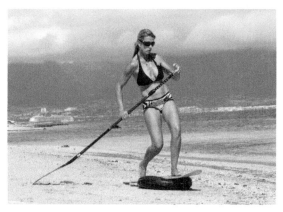
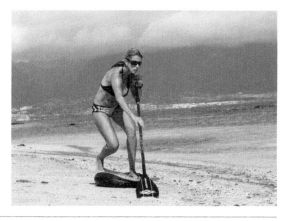

In real life, this is happening very fast—within a split second. So mimic the movement in the same manner. Remember as you're going through these exercises—don't follow the paddle with your eyes. Keep your gaze trained straight ahead.

PROGRESSION 3

The *Ultimate* in SUP Balance for Bracing

I have an actual video of this on You Tube on my Suzie Cooney channel should you wish to see this live. It's called "Stand Up Paddle Training Video Adding A New Dimension to Your SUP Performance." Check it out. *http://bit.ly/1fW724y*

Now that you've worked through the above progressions, it's time we get you as close as we can to the water's edge. I suggest you take all of the fins out of your SUP board for this and inflate the Inflate Indo Board Gigante Cushion to 80%. Be sure you're on grass or sand.

Place the cushion directly underneath the center of your SUP board, nubby side up. Make sure the board's not leaning from one rail to the other too much.

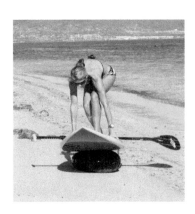

With paddle in hand, carefully tip the tail of your board on the ground and step on the back gently with your rear foot first and then the front foot apart and near the handle. Whoa. . . go easy. . . You will now be immediately in your preferred surf stance, and this is how we'll start.

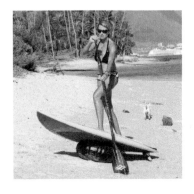
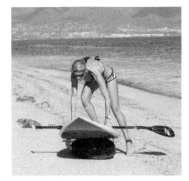
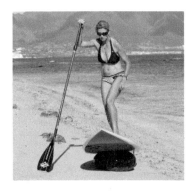

Find your sweet spot and just chill. You did it. Your eyes are still gazing forward and your paddle is still in this horizontal position. However, with the height of the board on top of the cushion you may get to practice a few strokes up there.

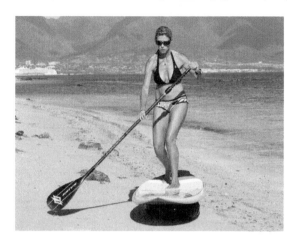 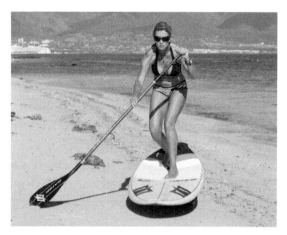

This is VERY tricky. Here we're going from surf stance to normal stance. Here's where you get to play and test your skill.

From this normal stance, step back as if you're going to catch a wave or turn around a buoy. If you start to fall, reach to the ground with your paddle but don't look where you plant it. Where did it end up? In front of you, to the side or behind you?

Now bring your foot back to the normal stance and repeat this at different tempos. Then bend your knees and get a bit lower. From this position do the same.

Step off and take a bow. Don't forget to replace your fins back in your board.

Get ready to pump it up in Chapter 4 as I give you all of my upper body training secrets to help you explode your paddling strength to an entirely new level!

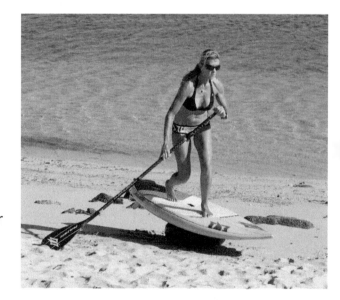

CHAPTER 4
How to Increase Your Upper Body Strength & Endurance for SUP

- Time to think lean, strong, light, and fast.
- Training your upper body for charging waves is different than training for distance or sprint racing.
- Working out your upper body requires a multi-faceted approach.
- Upper body strength and endurance building exercises: shoulders, back, chest, biceps, triceps.

Whether you're new to the sport of stand up paddling, preparing for an exciting Maui Maliko downwinder, or gearing up for a sprint race, having upper body paddling strength and endurance is critical to your success and enjoyment of the sport. I want you to have the ammunition and extreme body confidence you need to help you pass a competitor, make every wave, and dominate.

We'll focus on the upper half of your body: shoulders, chest, back, biceps and triceps. I will help you develop the entire shoulder complex, upper and lower back muscles, different points of the chest, and last, but not least, the triceps and biceps, which are also important.

Knowing how to train is also key to avoiding some of the overuse injuries that are common in SUP athletes. There is further information about that topic in Chapter 10.

✷ THINK LEAN, STRONG, LIGHT, AND FAST

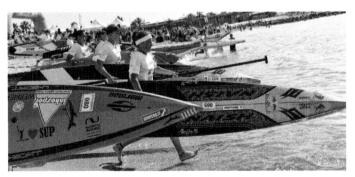

Manca Notar sprinting off the line

As a paddler and trainer I've noticed all types of bodies on the water. I've taken inventory at many start lines and observed that for the sport of SUP, no matter what type of event you're at, lean and light equal fast.

I'm reminded of one world champ, Manca Notar. She's amazing and is always strong from start to finish; she has a lightening fast cadence, but also shows her power in waves. Due to her conscious awareness of how she trains, she's able to do well in many disciplines of the sport.

And, speaking to this concept of light and lean, I recently had a former bodybuilder come to Maui and train with me to learn how to lean down and train in this manner for SUP. He was well aware that the years he spent putting on massive amounts of upper body bulk served him well for competition on the stage but actually slowed him down on the water.

In the time span of about seven months he made some major shifts in his diet and reduced the amount of heavy weight lifting that he was used to doing just so he could get faster and lighter on the water. He's seen a big improvement. He still has the same strength and power but now uses it just for explosive paddling sprints.

It's cool, when you look at the shoulder, front to top, top to back to see the "fine stripes," as I call them, of definition. You have to work hard for the stripes. To me that is the result of fine training of all the muscles in a proper manner for endurance. Having the perfect blend of power to push off the start, combined with the strength and endurance to maintain a steady pace throughout a race or event, is ideal.

My exercises and approach works. You'll be strong with the right amount of lean muscle for endurance but you'll also have the muscle strength for explosive paddling power.

BIG WAVE CHARGING VS. DISTANCE RACING

Training your upper body for charging waves is different than training for distance or sprint racing. Check out how strong Loch Eggers' chest is. Wow. This allows for some serious digging in to catch some serious big waves!

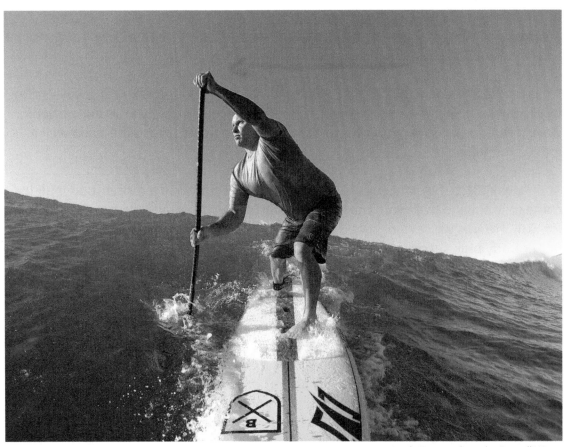

Loch Eggers photo by Darrell Wong

Stand up paddling on waves, big or small, requires you to use everything that you've been working on: core, balance and great reflexes. Now it's time for the upper body part. There's no doubt you should have a strong upper body and to know how to brace your weight on the paddle to help you carve and to prevent falls. You also need to have the strength to paddle into waves with 2-3 fast strokes or to get the hell out of dodge when a big set comes.

When you dig in hard to bury the blade to catch the wave of the day, do you have the juice in the shoulder to make the catch? What muscle do you feel first when the blade enters the water (besides the obliques)? I know the big guys may have an advantage to muscle through and that's cool, but soon enough the big muscles will give. Then what?

I have a saying when teaching people to get into waves. "If you're not catching that wave in 2-3 strokes, sit down or stop and wait for the next one." I notice, for sure, the difference between muscles I use to catch waves versus doing distance or cruising.

The most powerful "set" of shoulder muscles are of the rotator cuff, composed of the supraspinatus, infraspinatus, subscapularis, and teres minor. They, along with the tendons and ligaments, give you power when you need it most, but only if they are trained properly. Refer to Chapter 10 for an illustration of these muscles.

When you begin the series of exercises below, keep all the above in mind. Know that when you're training or strengthening any given muscle group you're also strengthening the supportive joints and tendons.

People often think if they have a wider blade on their paddle, they'll be able pull more water and catch more waves. While that could be partially true, you could also unknowingly be causing more stress on your shoulder. Because I train my shoulders properly I'm able to forgo a wider blade and rely on my strength. I don't get as tired as I have in the past when I was using a wider blade. More on that in Chapter 10.

WORKING OUT YOUR UPPER BODY REQUIRES A MULTI-FACETED APPROACH

It's amazing how often I see people overtraining their strongest upper body muscle group and under training their weakest link. Like the guys (some gals too) you see in the gym doing the same bicep curl in front of the mirror for hours. People love to train what they are good at because it's easy.

I used to train one of the fastest swimmers and record holder at the IRONMAN competition on the Big Island. His name is Jan Sibberson and he's from Germany. When he's on Maui to cool down and recover he stops in for some training and we have a blast.

He has a great saying that makes be laugh every time I say it but it's so true. In his deep German accent, he says, "Suzie, I have a chocolate side and a vinegar side. I want you to make my vinegar side like my chocolate side." He is hilarious and I totally get it.

I've applied this to my students and clients, too. It's like if we're super strong paddling on one side of the board because it's our chocolate side (the yummiest-the most comfortable), and the weaker side is the vinegar side.

So let's work on the vinegar parts and work on getting everything strong so your strokes are all chocolate.

UPPER BODY STRENGTH & ENDURANCE BUILDING EXERCISES

The following upper body exercises I've selected will increase your overall stand up paddling performance.

We're going to start with the shoulders, then the back, chest, biceps and triceps. Keeping in mind lean and mean and with the intention of training smart and in a balanced approach.

SHOULDER EXERCISES

Exercise 1:
STANDING TUBE CHOPS

You may have seen this one in my YouTube video called **Exercises for Stand Up Paddling to Help Avoid Common Injuries and Overuse Issues** *http://bit.ly/1VxnSXJ*

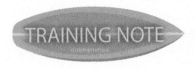

When performing this exercise, visualize delivering your blade to the water with a super-strong, driving force. If you were to slow down your stroke and think of the power coming down through the top of your shoulder, this is the one exercise that will increase it.

I'm starting with this exercise because first, it's my favorite and second, it delivers so many huge benefits to other muscles, including your chest, triceps, biceps, obliques, and lats. These muscles stabilize and assist your shoulder during execution of this exercise.

In a short amount of time you'll quickly gain noticeable strength and power.

SUGGESTED TRAINING EQUIPMENT

Light to heavy gauge tubing (I prefer tubes with cushioned handle), BOSU and/or Indo Board of choice, 24" Gigante Flo Cushion

SUGGESTED REPS/SETS

15-20 each side, 1-2 sets

MOVEMENT TEMPO/SPEED

Controlled with 1-2 second holds

PROGRESSION VARIABLES

Floor to BOSU, to Indo Board of choice to 24" Gigante Flo Cushion, medium gauge tube to heavy

PROGRESSION 1

Begin by securing tubing to a hook or something at least 2-3 feet above your head. Align your body perpendicular to the hook, with the right side of your body in line with the hook. Use your right hand to grab both handles of the tubing.

Next, bend your knees and place your left hand on your left thigh to steady yourself. Step a foot or so to your left to create some tension on the tube. Your right shoulder should be elevated and your elbow bent.

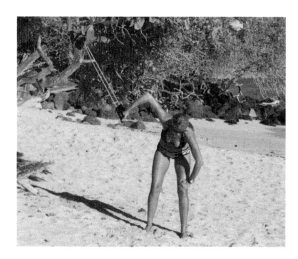 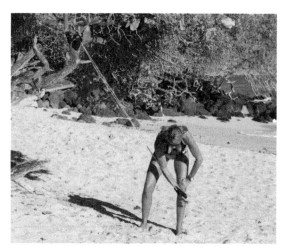

SUPER Important: Activate your right deep obliques and keep them engaged throughout the entire set. Now bring that handle in your right hand down and in front of the left knee and hold for one or two seconds. It's very important that you breathe out on every rep and keep your head down.

You should feel your chest muscles, biceps, and triceps also assisting you while your obliques are anchoring you. Remember, in Chapter 2 it was all about the obliques. Your core will always be a tremendous part of your strength for stand up paddling.

Return to start. Now the tube should have just a little slack in it and your elbow is up high and slightly bent. It's also important as you move on to the next rep that you keep your body hunkered down and low. Don't be tempted to bob up and down. Repeat on the left side.

NOTE: You may be weaker on the left side (if you're right handed) so you might want to step a bit closer towards the hook above. Don't force it. You'll get stronger as you train.

PROGRESSION 2

This progression is much harder. Now that you've got this down and it's nice and smooth, let's fire up the legs and core to the max by stepping up onto the BOSU with two feet. Now don't think you're too cool here by placing the BOSU farther out than where you were standing. You'll want to position the BOSU a smidge farther behind where you stood on the ground so your tube alignment remains true. These are tough; good luck.

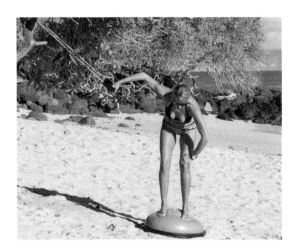 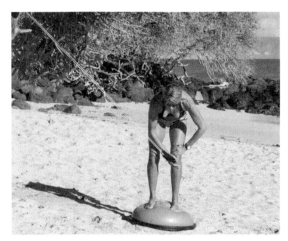

PROGRESSION 3

This is the most challenging. You'll be so fired up from head to toe you won't know your own name! Place your choice of Indo Board atop the 24 inch Gigante Flo Cushion with nubby side up. You'll feel everything shake down below but don't forget that your focus here is still on the shoulder muscle complex.

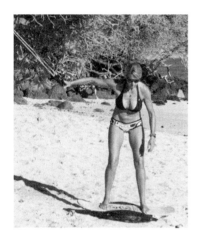 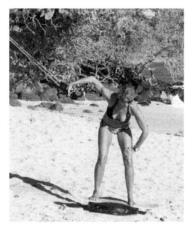 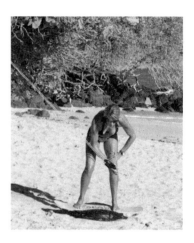

Exercise 2:
STABILITY BALL SEATED TUBE SHOULDER PULL DOWNS

This is an easier exercise but it's also hugely beneficial. I like this one because it's rhythmic and flowing, focusing on the shoulder, but you'll also get a little benefit for the core. Here we think of speed—lean and mean for sure.

People often tell me they want their shoulders to have stripes like mine. I blush and say, "Do these."

SUGGESTED TRAINING EQUIPMENT
Light to heavy gauge tubing (I prefer ones with cushioned handle.), firm stability ball

SUGGESTED REPS/SETS
15-20, 1-2 sets

MOVEMENT TEMPO/SPEED
Controlled with 1-2 second holds

PROGRESSION VARIABLES
Increase retraction hold of shoulder blades, light to medium gauge tubing, base of support (legs), stable to unstable, 2-1 leg

PROGRESSION 1

Use the same hook to affix your tubing that you did for the first exercise. Place the stability ball about two feet out from the pole or door to which you have affixed your tube and sit on top of it. With your legs bent at 90 degrees about shoulder width apart, grab the handles—one in each hand—and, with good posture, lean back slightly.

The tubing is now at about eye level and your elbows should be raised and bent. For now, pull the tubing back using a rowing action, taking a breath out for each rep. You can choose to keep this tempo flowing at a faster pace, or, to increase intensity, slightly retract your shoulder blades together and hold a second or two. You can experiment with this. You'll feel it, for sure.

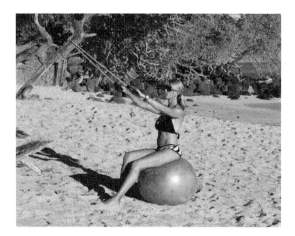
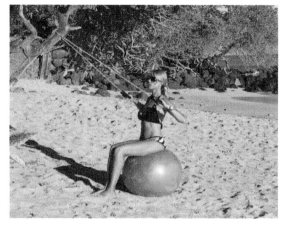

PROGRESSION 2

Bring your feet closer together to make your seating platform less stable. This will require you to use the deep core muscles to stabilize for a new set. More brainpower is required, as well, leading to more focused training.

PROGRESSION 3

To make this extremely challenging, you can now lift one leg up about 4 to 6 inches to reduce your base of support. Be careful that your hamstring does not cramp up.

Exercise 3:
STANDING SINGLE SHOULDER TUBE PRESSES

This exercise is also on my YouTube Channel Suzie Cooney which is titled: **Exercises for Stand Up Paddling to Help Avoid Common Overuse Injuries**
http://bit.ly/1VxnSXJ

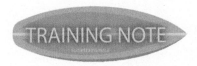

You'll notice I present you with a lot of exercises that require resistance bands. That's because, while using these, you are in constant check of the muscle force and tension relationship to your body.

When you train with machines, it's easy to lose the feel along the way. It's not to say that training on machines or with cable mechanisms is wrong; it's actually a nice variable to add. But if you want to really tune in, the tubing is great.

With this exercise we work one entire shoulder independently of the other. We incorporate all of the rotator cuff muscles to work together while the back and chest muscles support each rep.

This one takes practice and requires excellent form but is critical for good shoulder health and endurance on the water.

SUGGESTED TRAINING EQUIPMENT
Light to heavy gauge tubing (I prefer ones with cushioned handle)

SUGGESTED REPS/SETS
15-20, 1-2 sets

MOVEMENT TEMPO/SPEED
Slow and controlled with 1-2 second holds

PROGRESSION VARIABLES
Light to medium gauge tubing

Wrap your tubing around a pole. Let's start with the right shoulder. With your back toward the pole, place both handles in the right hand at about eye level, elbow up and bent. I call this "tango" position. Sort of like the dance.

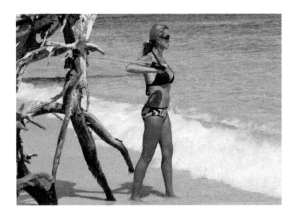 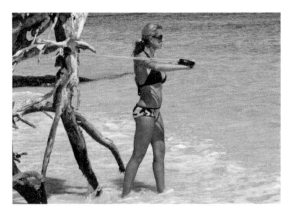

Your stance is staggered with a forward pelvic tilt. Your anchor is the rear glute of the leg behind you. Assume a nice tall posture with your shoulder blades squeezed gently in retraction. With your eyes trained forward, gently push the tubing out towards the front of you while keeping your shoulder blades together.

Only go as far as your shoulder will allow without losing the retraction. A reminder cue is if you keep your elbow up in the "tango" position you'll have an easier time maintaining it. This exercise should be smooth and controlled.

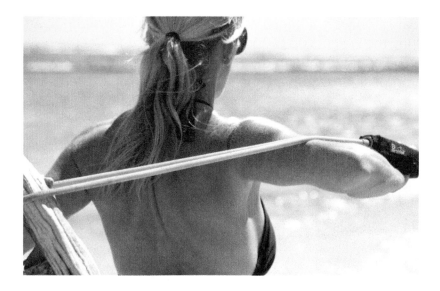

To increase difficulty, increase the gauge of the tubing used.

Exercise 4:
ALTERNATING DUMBBELL SHOULDER PRESSES

These are your standard shoulder presses but I prefer to do these as alternating presses in order to avoid straining the neck and to avoid any forward jutting of the head. Weights do have a role in your training—to build muscle mass and to create more force production delivery to the paddle as you enter the blade.

SUGGESTED TRAINING EQUIPMENT
Weights 5-12 pounds, bench or stability ball

SUGGESTED REPS/SETS
15-20, (30-40 total) 1-2 sets

MOVEMENT TEMPO/SPEED
Controlled with good form

PROGRESSION VARIABLES
Increase weight

Sit on top of the stability ball or on weight bench with your feet shoulder width apart and a nice, tall posture. Bring the weights up to shoulder level, palms facing the mirror (or outward). Press the right hand up to the ceiling, breathing out. Once you return the weight to the start position, complete the same sequence on the left side.

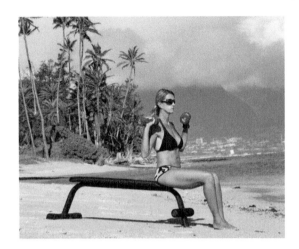 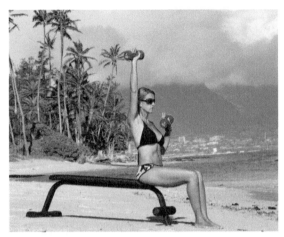

As you press up I want you think of all the power coming up through the shoulder to the ceiling. Feel it through the entire shoulder complex.

Only increase weight if your form is solid.

Exercise 5:
PADDLE BREAKS ON STABILITY BALL

This one is very popular, and is highlighted in my Suzie Cooney YouTube Channel as **How to Bring More Power to the Blade**. *http://bit.ly/1OazefO*

People love this one and tell me they feel such an increase in power when they paddle after doing just a few sets of these.

Talk about a driving force of power transferred from the top of deltoid to the blade, to the water? This one is killer and very challenging. It also requires incredible attention to your core, thighs and legs. You could also consider this as a balance challenge.

SUGGESTED TRAINING EQUIPMENT
Light to heavy gauge tubing, firm stability ball

SUGGESTED REPS/SETS
15-20, 1-2 sets

MOVEMENT TEMPO/SPEED
Controlled with good form, 1-3 second hold

PROGRESSION VARIABLES
Increase tubing gauge, increase hold time, move feet closer together

PROGRESSION 1

Secure the resistance tube around or to a sturdy object the height of the stability ball or just a bit higher. Sit on top of the stability ball. Hold the tubing in each hand, with your hands behind you and slowly move your feet forward so your knees are bent into a 90 degree angle. Place your feet firmly on the ground, toes pointed forward with neck and shoulders on the stability ball. The tubing should now be slightly above your head, arms extended behind you and feet less than shoulder width apart.

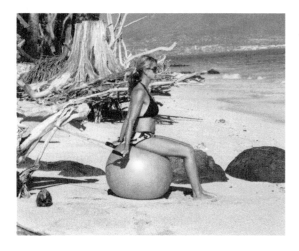 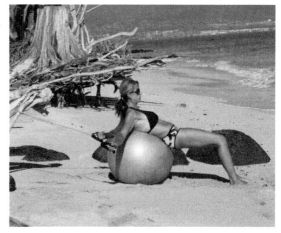

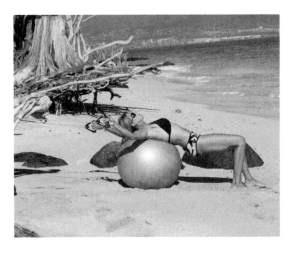 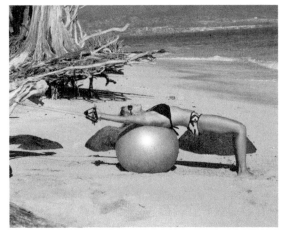

Next, without gripping the handles too tightly, pull the tubing towards your knees. To help keep you stable on the ball, try and engage your core muscles such as your abs and glutes as you begin and complete each rep. Avoid squeezing the glutes too much so you don't cramp.

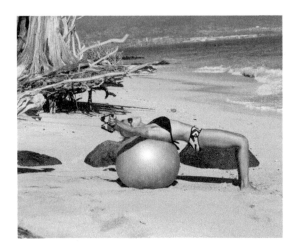 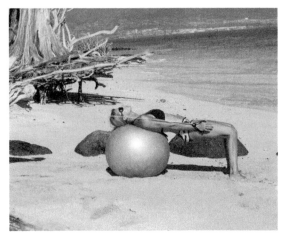

With each rep, breathe out. Inhale as you return. Because you can't see yourself performing this exercise in the mirror, it's also considered a great proprioceptive or brain exercise as well. Good balance and a strong core helps.

PROGRESSION 2

To increase the challenge, bring your feet closer together and repeat the movement described above. You will really have to concentrate on this transition.

Exercise 6:
STANDING PRONE PADDLE TUBE PRESSES

You may have seen this one in my M20 video as it was my favorite to "keep the rust" off the muscles before the big day. I love this, as I can adjust the effort and intensity on the fly. An added bonus of this one is the cardio benefit. Also, if you do it correctly, your core and deep abdominal muscles get a blast too. Any time you're in the "prone" position your heart will work four times harder.

Although the emphasis is the shoulders, you'll feel your lats or latissimus dorsi fire as you pull the tubing toward you. This feels awesome!

Our focus is smooth padding and a smooth exercise. While I do this exercise, I literally think of and visualize every rep as a paddle stroke.

SUGGESTED TRAINING EQUIPMENT
Light to heavy gauge tubing

SUGGESTED REPS/SETS
20-25, 1-3 sets, timed sets: 30 seconds to 2 minutes

MOVEMENT TEMPO/SPEED
Controlled with good form, slow to fast as tension allows

PROGRESSION VARIABLES
Increase tubing gauge, hold 1-2 seconds after each rep, 1 leg, unstable platform BOSU, half foam roller, Indo Board with Gigante Flo Cushion

---

PROGRESSION 1

Secure tubing, hip high, around a sturdy object. Face the sturdy object, while holding the tubing in each hand, and step away from the object securing tubing. Place your feet together, knees bent, with a slight hinge, bent over at the hips, and hold the tubing with enough tension to allow for a full-length motion above your head past your thighs. Adjust the distance accordingly to allow for a full repetition, and, most importantly, keep your head in a neutral position (not tilted forward or backward).

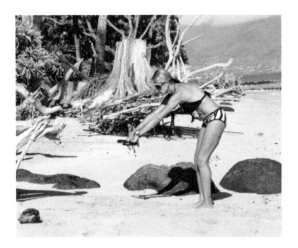 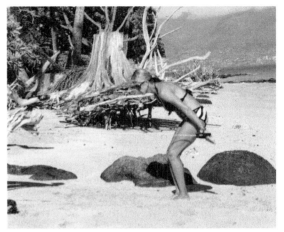

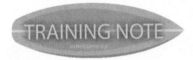

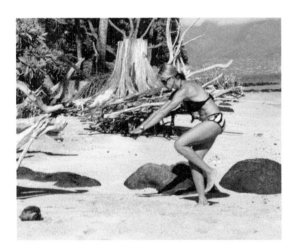 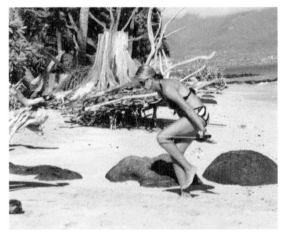

Now this is work, so pace yourself, otherwise your form will suffer. Your last rep should be as good as your first with every set. Find a rhythm that you can maintain with a breath out for each rep.

Another tip is to make sure that with each rep you really engage the deep muscles of your core as an anchor so you can keep the focus on the shoulders.

As your fitness and strength increases you may advance to a heavier gauge tube.

PROGRESSION 2

These are incredibly challenging. Changing the platform from the floor to an unstable platform takes this to an entire new level. This progression is almost like a total body conditioning exercise so be sure, again, to keep the emphasis on the shoulder complex. You may need to switch to a tube with less resistance so you can perform each rep with good form. These are listed in order of difficulty, easiest to most challenging.

BOSU: You may need to move tubing up about one foot to accommodate for the height of the BOSU. Step up with two feet and space your feet less than shoulder width apart. Find the right tension, keep your head in neutral position, and go for it.

Half foam roller: Place foam horizontally and step on with two feet and knees bent. Go easy, find your sweet spot, and good luck!

Indo Board Pro Kicktail and 24" Gigante Flo Cushion: This could rock your world from shoulders to legs, so go easy. Any Indo Board will do and remember, less air in the cushion offers more 4 way water-like action.

With nubby side up, position cushion at similar distance as you did with the BOSU above, take your board and place it horizontally, straight and centered. Immediately bend your knees as you step on with two feet—a bit wider this time than shoulder width apart—and as you get better to the overall action, you can bring them together.

BACK EXERCISES

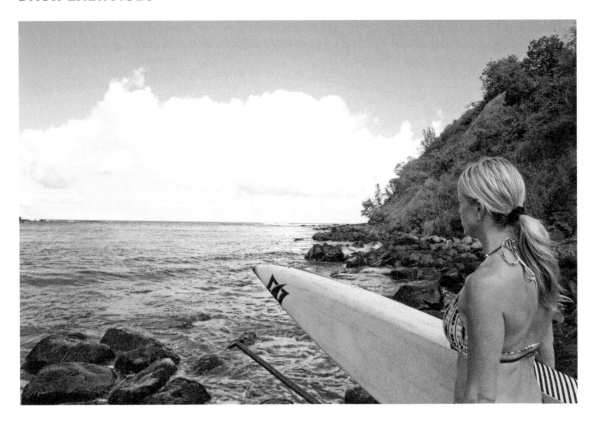

"Paddler's got back." Sorry, I could not resist. I guess this gets me because I started my modeling career way *back* as a "back" model at 18 for the bathing suit company Barely Legal. What I can say?

The back muscles are important and act as stabilizing muscles to help you execute each stroke. They also keep you upright for all types of stand up padding. The upper and lower back muscles must be strong and carry a tremendous load—especially during distance paddling. You can see an illustration of the back muscles in Chapter 10.

Your back muscles support the shoulder complex and core, allowing you to connect one stroke one after the other. I remember my lower back was getting sore on the M2O crossing when we hit the dreaded patch of currents that were backwashing off Oahu. I felt like I wasn't moving and, wow, the stress of that seemed to go right to my weak part.

When you paddle surf, your lower back is twisting with your hips as you carve, and the upper back muscles assist your shoulder to plant your paddle blade along the wall.

One very important concept you'll need to understand for some of these exercises is the art of what I have coined "holding the money" or having the ability to keep your shoulder blades of the back tight and together all throughout a full repetition. If you aren't strong enough to hold the money and you're not Jerry Maguire who can *show* you the money, you go broke and your form and paddle stroke go to crap.

Exercise 1:
STANDING 1-ARMED ROWS LAWNMOWERS

This exercise will strengthen the trapezius and minor and major rhomboids. This is also referred to as a standing row.

You are the machine that stabilizes all throughout this weighted back exercise.

SUGGESTED TRAINING EQUIPMENT
5-25 pound dumbbells

SUGGESTED REPS/SETS
12-15, 1-2 sets

MOVEMENT TEMPO/SPEED
Controlled with good form

PROGRESSION VARIABLES
Increase dumbbell weight

Start with a dumbbell weight that's comfortable for a full set. Starting with the right side bring your left leg forward into a slight lunge with a bent knee. Lean forward at the waist and hips and rest your left forearm on the thigh of your left leg. Keep your head and neck in a neutral position. Your right leg should be a bit straighter with your right foot pointed to the right.

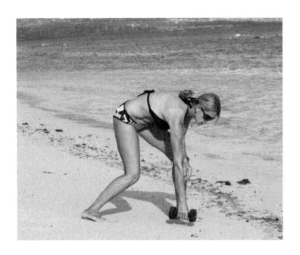 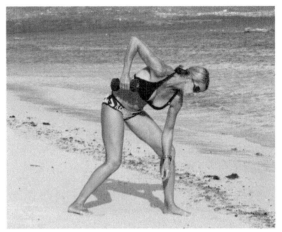

Holding the dumbbell in your right hand, let the weight rest on the floor. Engage your core by drawing in your stomach to the front of your spine, and pull your elbow up toward the ceiling without raising your body up. Breathe out. Return and repeat. Then do the same for the left side.

Exercise 2:
STABILITY BALL SEATED TUBE ROWS

This is where you need to "hold the money" and learn about assuming and maintaining the position of retraction. So first let's practice this concept by having you sit on the stability ball in good posture. Keep shoulders back, pinching your shoulder blades behind you without allowing your trapezius to rise up to your ears or allowing the scalenes, or your front neck muscles, to strain. Make sure you can breathe while you do this.

This is difficult to grasp at first, but you must know how to do this well before we go on. Another visual would be for you to imagine you are squeezing your shoulder blades together and pressing them down into your back pockets. Got it so far? You have to really concentrate.

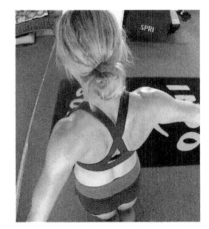

SUGGESTED TRAINING EQUIPMENT
Light to heavy gauge tubing, firm stability ball

SUGGESTED REPS/SETS
15-20, 1-2 sets

MOVEMENT TEMPO/SPEED
Slow and controlled with good form, 1-3 second hold

PROGRESSION VARIABLES
Increase tubing gauge feet closer together, 2-1 leg

PROGRESSION 1

Begin by securing the tubing around a sturdy object and sit up nice and tall on a firm stability ball. To start, sit with your feet about hip width apart and bent at a 90 degree angle. You'll want tension on the resistance tubing but not too much at first. Sit with your eyes forward, elbows held close to your ribcage and bent at 90 degrees, with your back and shoulder blades in retraction or holding the money. Note: Don't death grip the handles so you don't get forearm pump.

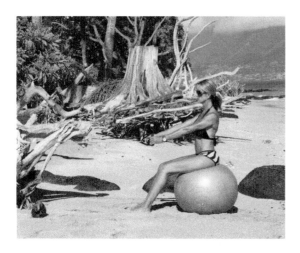 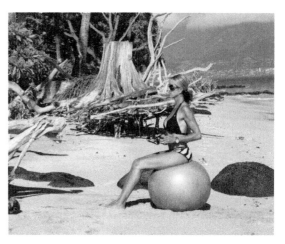

Slowly pull the handles towards your body, as this range of motion is slight, and hold the money. Pinch gently and hold for a count of at least two seconds. Don't hold your breath and use a controlled motion—it's a small return to start. Again, this repetition and movement is small. Don't allow your hand and elbows to return too far forward in front of your body. If you do, you'll drop the money!

PROGRESSION 2

As you've probably noticed, it's not easy to control the upper back motion. As you progress, sitting with your feet close together changes it up a bit. Now your core muscles need to keep you still as you complete each repetition.

PROGRESSION 3

This one is tricky. You must be careful to not let your glutes on the supporting leg take over. Assume the same position as above in Progression 1 with great form and retraction the main emphasis.

Carefully lift the right leg about 3-4 inches up off the floor and attempt a few smooth repetitions. The focus is still the back, so be careful. Your core is probably firing, which is great, and your thigh is burning, but it's all about the back. Good luck.

Exercise 3:
STABILITY BALL LOWER BACK EXTENSIONS

Paddling can definitely take a toll on the lower back sometimes, as the back helps keep you upright. When it comes to training it for stand up paddling, I have selected this simple lower back exercise because it requires you to be the machine—like most of the exercises in this book.

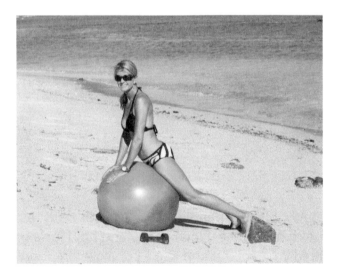

You will need your core, especially your glutes, to fire and support you all throughout each rep and set.

SUGGESTED TRAINING EQUIPMENT
Firm stability ball

SUGGESTED REPS/SETS
15-20, 1-2 sets

MOVEMENT TEMPO/SPEED
Controlled with good form, 1-3 second hold

PROGRESSION VARIABLES
Supported, weighted

PROGRESSION 1

Supported

Select a clear space near a base of a wall or heavy item like a couch or treadmill. Lie prone on the ball with hips forward. Brace your feet against the wall or object with your knees slightly bent and shoulder width apart.

There are two different positions you can attempt. The first one may help you steady yourself on the ball and the second one requires a bit more skill.

Position One: Cross arms in front of shoulders. Lift your chest and torso off of ball by arching your lower back. Squeeze your glutes to help you maintain good form. As you get to the top of the motion, breathe out. Return and lower torso and chest to ball. Repeat.

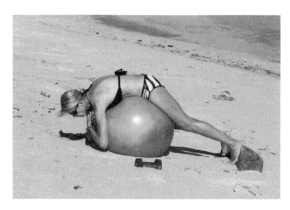 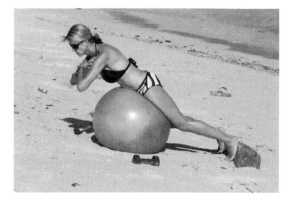

Position Two: Bend your elbows and place your hands behind your head, fingers spread wide, not locked together. Lower your chest and torso down over the ball, contract your glutes and rise up slowly with a big breath out.

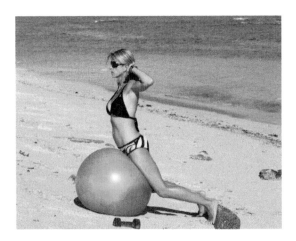

PROGRESSION 2

Supported with weight

Select a weight, such as an 8-12 pound dumbbell and hold onto each end as you're bent over the ball. Hold the dumbbell close to your body, contract your glutes for additional lower back support and rise up as you did in Progression 1. Exhale.

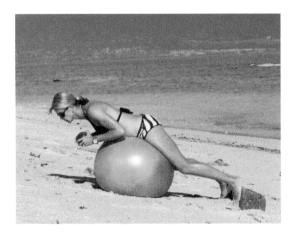 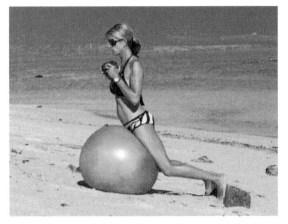

PROGRESSION 3

Unsupported with and without weight

This position really requires a bit more concentration and strength. Now we will take away your feet from the sturdy object so you will have to rely on our entire body. This will also require you to call upon the deeper core muscles to help you stabilize on the ball.

Best to place stability ball on top of a carpet, mat, or sticky yoga mat that allows you to grip with your toes. (Note: If on carpet or mat, best to perform this with shoes on. If you're on a sticky yoga mat, you can try this barefoot.) Assume the same prone position as you did in Progression 1 above with your feet a *bit wider* behind you than the original exercise. By having your feet wider, you can keep the ball steady throughout the exercise. Contract your glutes and begin the rep of your desire. You can perform this with arms crossed in front of you or try with your elbows bent behind you—first without weights, and then maybe adding a dumbbell for an extra challenge.

Exercise 4:
STANDING 2 ARM DUMBBELL BACK ROWS

This next back exercise is also in the prone, or bent over, position and will get the heart going. Remember anything you do while in the prone position challenges the heart four times of anything you do in the upright position.

I like this exercise because I believe it lends great base power to your stroke. It's like the bass guitar in a band adding that extra something special to wow the crowd. Well, this is like that. This will give your back muscles a strong base of strength to execute amazing paddling. We can also adjust the exercise to allow for endurance strength training of the back as well. You would simply reduce the dumbbell weight and increase the tempo.

For an added twist on the challenge factor you can place one of your feet onto an unstable platform to challenge your footing as you perform each rep. See Progressions below.

SUGGESTED TRAINING EQUIPMENT

Dumbbells 5-15 pounds, BOSU, half foam roller, Indo Board Pro Kicktail, Gigante Flo Cushion

SUGGESTED REPS/SETS

12-15, 1-2 sets

MOVEMENT TEMPO/SPEED

Moderate, controlled with good form, 1-3 second hold

PROGRESSION VARIABLES

Increase weight, increase tempo, place foot on unstable platform

PROGRESSION 1

Stand with a staggered stance about three feet apart and bend over at the hip. Keep your head in a neutral position and, with a dumbbell in each hand, allow the weights to rest low near your feet. Pull both weights up together toward your chest, and, at the top of the movement, gently pinch our shoulder blades together as a cue to help you maintain good form. You don't need to squeeze hard. Breathe out.

What I like to do is switch feet in my stance at about rep number ten or on my second set. Increase weight accordingly.

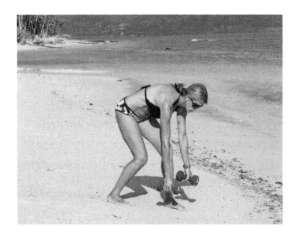 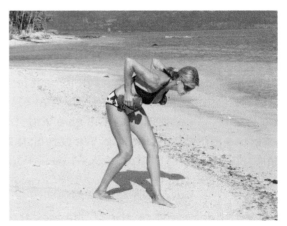

PROGRESSION 2

As you've learned by now you can really change up the variables in these exercises by adding a balance component. You'll notice added stress to your leg so that's a good thing, but remember to keep focused on the back muscles throughout each set.

I've listed the gear in the order in my suggested order from least to most challenging. Below are some photos so you can see what they all look like.

First, the BOSU: Place the arch of one foot directly on top of the BOSU. With your other leg behind you on the floor, turn out that foot a bit at an angle for added support. Now begin as you would in Progression 1. Feeling your leg fire up a bit? Very cool. You're doing it right.

Next, place your foot on the half foam roller and give this a try. It's a different kind of challenge, and, again you'll feel the muscles in the foot, ankle, and leg fire.

The best for last is the Gigante Flo Cushion and any Indo Board. Note that the Pro Kicktail, due to its narrowness, offers an intense leg challenge. This time you'll place your foot vertical and in the center of the board with the board direction horizontally. Be careful of placing too much weight on there, as we don't want to forget this is a back exercise. Good luck and have fun.

Exercise 5:
STANDING TRX BACK ROWS

Remember that your strong upper back is going to help your overall performance so you're not that all arm paddler you see sometimes inching forward in the water, t-rex arms and all. This is a good one but requires lots of brainpower. You're getting stronger with each exercise you perform to be a stronger stand up paddler. So, as hard as this might get, that is why you're here with me.

We could go a little nuts here and ramp up the balance challenge but I want to keep the focus of this exercise on strength.

Now that you're a pro at "holding the money" let's see how much cash you can keep in that strong upper back region. Here it's key to start practicing the skill of visualization training. We'll go deeper on that in Chapter 7. Since you can't "see" the muscle your training you'll use your imagination to ensure good form.

I have to mention that I wish this TRX Rip Trainer bar was lighter in weight overall, but since it does take on a lot of torque and tension I get they had to make it heavy duty to stand up to the test. Having this bar can lead to forearm pump or burn so keep that in mind.

SUGGESTED TRAINING EQUIPMENT
TRX Rip Trainer, heavy gauge cord, BOSU

SUGGESTED REPS/SETS
15-20, 1-2 sets

MOVEMENT TEMPO/SPEED
Controlled with good form, slow to fast, 1-2 second hold

PROGRESSION VARIABLES
Speed/tempo change, BOSU

PROGRESSION 1

Secure your TRX RIP Trainer chest-high around a pole or use the door jam accessory that came with your kit. Make sure one hand is in the safety loop and place your hands at opposite ends of the bar, holding it up to chest level.

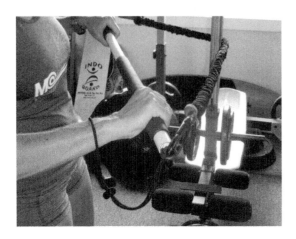
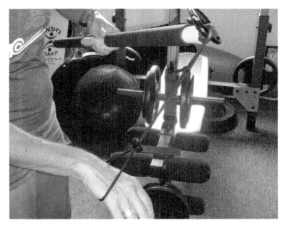

Assume a staggered stance position with elbows up at shoulder height. To help my clients maintain good form, I call this the "tango" position. Grab the Rip Trainer on opposite ends, be sure the bar is screwed tight and hold it at chest high. Relax your upper shoulders, especially the traps or trapezium, and don't allow the front of your neck to strain. Step away from pole or door to create tension on the cord.

Stay with me. Now, if you think it couldn't get more exciting, let's get a pelvic tilt going forward so you don't over arch your lower back. Squeeze the butt muscle of the back supporting leg.

"Hold the money" all throughout each set and only perform each repetition to the extent to which you will not drop your change and maintain excellent form.

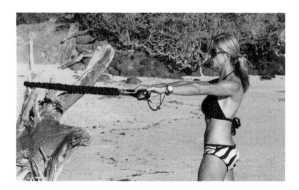 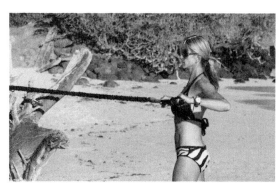

While shoulder blades are in retraction, you're in the tango-staggered stance, with eyes and head forward. Pull the Rip Trainer towards your chest for one rep and exhale out. To increase the intensity hold each rep for a count of two seconds. This movement is very small. Return to start position and repeat.

You can experiment with speed of reps and tension.

Exercise 6:
STANDING 2 ARM TUBE BACK ROWS

If you think you've got money invested in your back now, hold on to your paddle. Here we go again with the "hold the money" fun. Have my banker call your banker and we'll go for a paddle. These also make your back super strong and sexy!

With all that you know about your back and how important it is to support your whole body, let's keep going. You will definitely feel this exercise a day or two after.

SUGGESTED TRAINING EQUIPMENT
Light to heavy gauge tubing, firm stability ball

SUGGESTED REPS/SETS
15-20, 1-2 sets

MOVEMENT TEMPO/SPEED
Controlled with good form, 1-3 second hold

PROGRESSION VARIABLES
Increase tubing gauge, increase hold time

Begin by putting resistance tube at about chest high around pole or secure in door jam if you have the accessory to do so. You will now almost do the same thing that you did in Exercise 3 above but this time you'll have your back to the pole or door.

Grab the handles, holding one in each hand. Then turn around and face the opposite direction as the pole. (See photo.) Assume a staggered stance with a pelvic tilt forward, arms up in tango position, shoulder blades in retraction, and with your eyes looking forward. Press the tubing out with your back muscles and hold the money. Exhale your breath out.

Like the TRX Rip Trainer exercise, you have to imagine "seeing" the muscles of your back hard at work. This is not an arm or chest exercise, but they definitely do assist and you'll feel the pectoral muscles working too. However, stay focused on the back.

Your movement is only as far as you can press the tube with good form and without dropping the money; this is your first rep. Return in a slow and controlled manner to start. These are killer if you do them right.

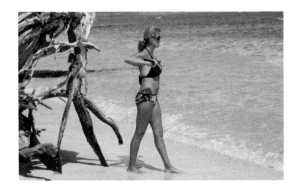 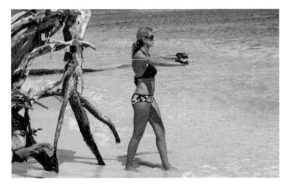

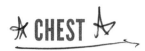 CHEST

Like your back, the chest is a key muscle group that obviously houses a great deal of power. It's also important in stabilizing your core and acts as the structural chamber of your body while your paddling. The main muscles of the chest are called the pectoralis major and minor.

In the chest there is plenty of ammunition that fires and extends to and through your shoulders to the blade and to the water at that moment in time when you are digging hard to catch a wave, or, just the opposite, paddling away from a wave that is about to crush you!

Right before the start of a sprint the muscles of the chest add that extra juice you need to lift that board forward and out of the water in order to get in the top five, fast.

A strong chest also helps to keep your body upright for good posture while you paddle. I'd like to get back to the thought of the lean and mean concept. If you're already a huge barrel of chest thunder, good for you, but you don't want to over train what you're already blessed with. Instead, maybe go easy and build your endurance here. You can refer to Chapter 9 to learn more.

If you'd like to have more strength and power for every stroke, let's do this.

Exercise 1:
STANDARD / KNEE BENT PUSH UPS

Let's get this done with no whining. I want you to learn to love push ups. This was my weapon of choice in my training arsenal before the M2O. I would do twenty a day for two months because I knew getting up and down off my board if I fell could make me tired. And I knew I would need every ounce of extra power to conserve energy getting on and off the escort boat.

Push ups work the pectoral muscles and also strengthen the shoulders, triceps and core.

If you haven't noticed, my arms are super long, and, because of that, I have a harder time doing a standard push up. The peeps that have a shorter wingspan have a huge advantage. I'm not making excuses; it's an anatomical fact. So I would do knee bent with a clap in between. Listen, I needed all the applause I could get to keep me motivated.

SUGGESTED TRAINING EQUIPMENT
Perfect push up bars (no swivel preferred), training mat, hard medicine ball, BOSU

SUGGESTED REPS/SETS
10-15, 1-2 sets

MOVEMENT TEMPO/SPEED
Controlled with good form, 1-3 second hold

PROGRESSION VARIABLES
Change position of hands, 1 leg off the ground, add a clap, on medicine ball, 2-1 arm

PROGRESSION 1

Knee Bent

You can also place hands on a bench. Begin by kneeling on the mat with both knees shoulder width apart. Place hands (see photo) in front of you, palms-down, on the floor, approximately shoulder width apart. They should be about next to your shoulders, with your elbows pointed towards your feet behind you. Your head and neck should be held in a neutral state. Engage your core muscles and lower your body to the ground. Don't allow your butt to fly into the air, and bring your chin towards the ground. Slowly push up to your start position and repeat. Maintain a straight back and keep tempo smooth and controlled. Push a big breath out. Do not allow your head to drop or jut forward.

PROGRESSION 2

Standard Push up

Begin in a plank position on the floor with your feet together and hands slightly wider than shoulder-width apart. Engage your core muscles. Keeping your back flat and head neutral. Slowly lower your body to the floor. If you can't make it all the way (as if your chin is touching the floor), push back up to starting position. Do not allow your head to drop or jut forward or let your hips sag. Exhale a big breath out.

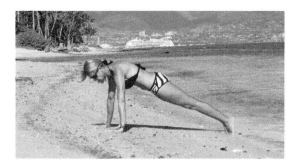 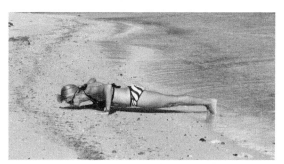

Various hand positions: You can also change up the standard push up with different hand positions underneath you. For example, the triangle position with hands wider or hands closer to the interior of your chest. Find the right one for you and mix it up. Each unique angle or position offers different types stress to the tricep and bicep region and the others more stress on the chest. These types of variable changes do provide continuous stress to the chest, which is the goal.

You can also try the perfect push up bars as they don't stress your wrists as badly as placing your hands flat on the ground. For different variations you can also change the angle or width of these.

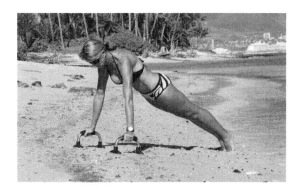 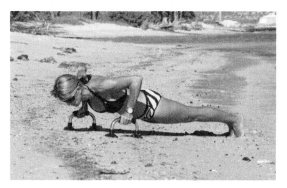

The triangle position will elicit more bicep action. Placing the hands in a wider position causes the pectoral walls to really come into play. With the hands closer to the inside of your chest your triceps might scream louder. It's all good!

Lastly, you can also place your feet on top of a BOSU to mix things up and recruit the core muscles at a higher level.

PROGRESSION 3

1 leg push up

Level of difficulty: *"very."* Think you're tough? Good luck on this one. Since we'll be firing up the glute and hamstrings on this as well, go easy so you don't get an unexpected cramp.

Assume plank position as in Progression 2. Lift one leg off the ground before you lower yourself down to the floor. Make sure that your form is not compromised in any way. Do half of your set with one leg up then switch to the other.

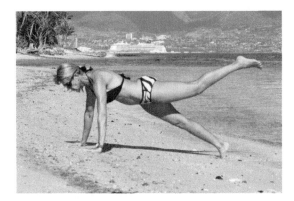 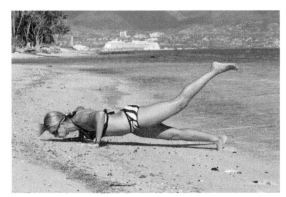

PROGRESSION 4

BOSU 1 Arm, 1 leg

This exercise rocks and really surprises most, as it's an incredible target directly to the chest but just one side at a time. You can modify this one by doing it on your knees just as in Progression 1. You may want to pace yourself and do a split of say five on one side and then five on the other. You can also incorporate the one leg variable as well.

First, place BOSU on the ground dome side up. Place your right hand centered on top and the other hand on the ground a little wider than shoulder-width apart. In the push up plank position lower your body toward the ground. You will place most the emphasis on your left chest wall as the right hand must stabilize each repetition.

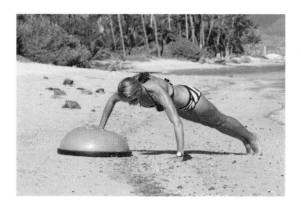
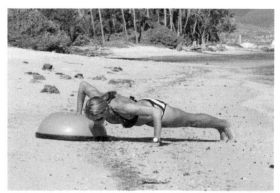

PROGRESSION 5

Push ups on Medicine Ball 2-1 arm, 1 leg, toes on BOSU

As always, I'm saving the best and most difficult for last. This is actually quite fun. I'll let you define "fun." I like it because you have to keep the medicine ball still. This takes focus and all the foundations of good form to execute properly. Your core muscles will also be activating at a much higher capacity.

Now that you're the push up champ of the SUP universe, take all you know and place two hands in a sort of tight triangle on a firm medicine ball with feet spread shoulder-width behind you.

Start in the standard plank push up position and lower your chest to the medicine ball, then press back up, breathing out. Stabilize and repeat. Keep your back straight and don't allow your head to fall or jut forward or let hips sag.

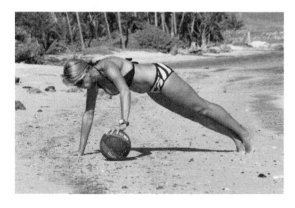
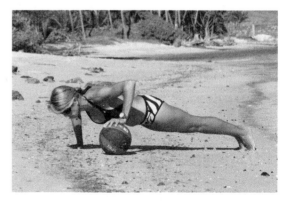

Next, place one hand on the medicine ball and one on the ground and assume standard push up position. This is similar to Progression 4 with the BOSU. Don't let the ball move and allow your core to help you. You can increase the challenge by moving your feet closer together.

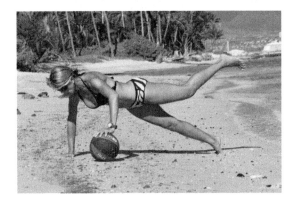 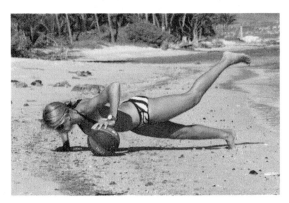

Exercise 2:
BENCH DUMBBELL PRESS

Here we target the chest with the bench supporting you. I like using a bench because it allows you to support your neck and lower back. You're then able to increase your load safely.

SUGGESTED TRAINING EQUIPMENT
Weight bench, dumbbells 5-20 pounds

SUGGESTED REPS/SETS
12-20, 1-3 sets

MOVEMENT TEMPO/SPEED
Controlled with good form

PROGRESSION VARIABLES
2-Arm, alternating arms, pec flys and standard presses, add weight accordingly

Place your head and shoulders on the bench. I like to place my feet on the bench to assure a flat back so I don't strain my lower back. Try it. Start with both weights on your chest and press them together toward the ceiling, breathing out on the way up. Return just below or at breast line. Repeat.

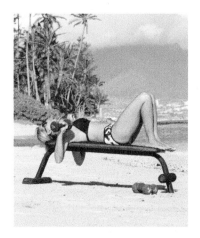 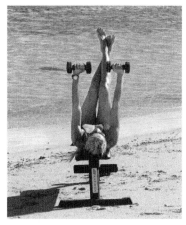 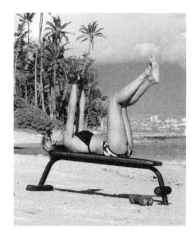

Be sure to keep weights over your chest and not your face, all the while maintaining a good bridge. Don't allow your lower back to arch. Before you progress to a heavier weight make sure both arms are working together in unison and make sure your neck never lifts off the bench.

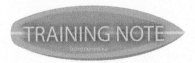 *Another trick I like to do to allow for a "deeper" start position of weights is to bring my legs up and cross my ankles at the top.*

You can change this up by alternating each arm or you can do pec flys, which allow for a nice stretch on the way down. Then you activate the chest wall to press back to start. Remember to breathe out on return to start.

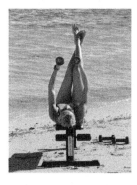 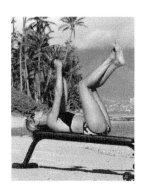 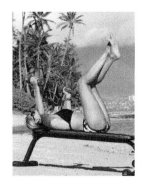 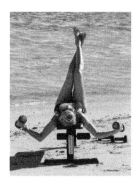

Exercise 3:
TRX RIP TRAINER CHEST PRESSES

This is similar to the back exercise outlined earlier in the chapter but this time you step inside the Rip Trainer. This requires you to again be the machine. In addition to the chest, it also targets the shoulders and back as those muscles help stabilize you throughout the movement.

SUGGESTED TRAINING EQUIPMENT
TRX Rip Trainer, heavy cord

SUGGESTED REPS/SETS
15-20, 1-2 sets

MOVEMENT TEMPO/SPEED
Controlled with good form, 1-3 second hold

PROGRESSION VARIABLES
Change up the tempo and tension

Secure your TRX RIP Trainer at about chest height around a pole or use the door jam accessory that came with your kit. Make sure one hand is in the safety loop and place one hand at each end of the bar. Hold it up to chest level and step inside the bar. (See photos on next page.)

Have the Rip Trainer resting on your chest and assume a staggered stance position with elbows up at shoulder height. Let's tango with a secure pelvic tilt. Grab the Rip Trainer on opposite ends; be sure the bar is screwed tight and hold it up at chest height.

Relax your upper shoulders, especially the traps or trapezium, and don't allow the front of your neck to strain. Step away from pole or door to create some decent tension on the cord.

Now press the Rip Trainer away from your chest and extend your arms straight out in front and exhale. Be sure not to grip too tight and pump the forearms.

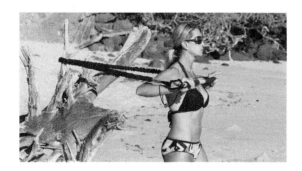 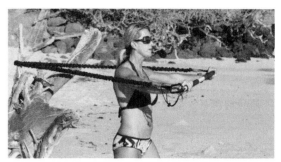

BICEPS

I joke I've been training my biceps hard since I was 16. It's actually no joke. I was curling 15-20 pounds single arm to be able to lift a dirt bike off myself and to be able to transport, by myself, a huge old 12 foot plastic windsurf board around that weighed A LOT and was longer than my car.

For stand up paddling the strength of your biceps—again plural like the triceps—is more important than you might think. The biceps muscle is actually composed of two muscles not one, as many people think. Its function allows your elbow to bend and create tremendous force between the elbow and shoulder. The biceps also assist in the rotation of your wrist and elbow to twist the paddle as the blade exits the water.

And the obvious is true, by having stronger, maybe a little bigger, biceps you can more forcefully explode of the start. Should you get into to real trouble, just flexing might scare off a competitor—or at least make them nervous!

SUGGESTED TRAINING EQUIPMENT
Dumbbells 5-20 pounds, weight bench or chair, resistance tubing, half BOSU, Gigante Cushion with Indo Board any board of choice

SUGGESTED REPS/SETS
12-20, 1-2 sets

MOVEMENT TEMPO/SPEED
Controlled with good form

PROGRESSION VARIABLES
Regular, hammer, 2-1 Arm, add weight accordingly, standing or seated, alternating, 2-1 leg, unstable platform

Exercise 1:
BASIC CURLS REGULAR & HAMMER

PROGRESSION 1

The basic curl is simple. I suggest to first perfect your form while seated on bench. Select a weight you can manage smoothly without straining. Sit with good posture and a tall spine, shoulders back, chest out and shoulders in slight retraction, elbows tight to rib cage.

To perform a regular curl, hold the dumbbells with your palms facing the mirror (or away from you) and bring the weight up towards your bicep. Do not keep a death grip on them. Return to bottom and repeat. Don't allow your head to jut forward or your body to rock. If you do either one of these things you're lifting too much and you need to pick up smaller weights.

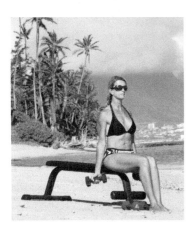 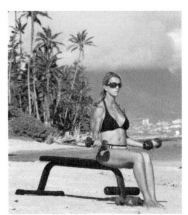 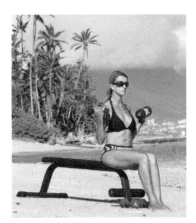

Now to target the head of the bicep, specifically the brachioradialis, which is the stronger flexor of the elbow; you'll perform a "hammer" curl.

Assume the same, seated position as in Progression 1 with perfect posture. Grab the dumbbells just below the bulk of weight with your palms turned inward. Lower the weights to your side and bring them up toward your bicep muscle. That is a hammer curl.

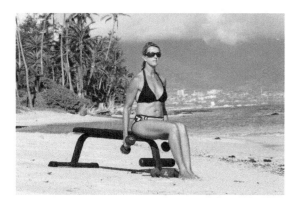 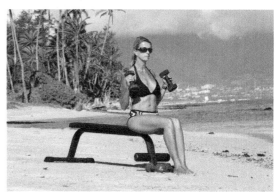

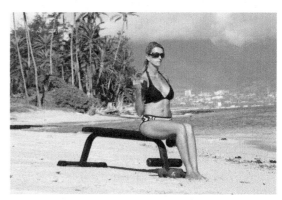

Variable note: You can perform two at the same time or do alternating reps. If you want to go up in weight sometimes alternating will serve you best.

PROGRESSION 2

This is simple. Simply doing these standing up will take a bit more focus and strength. You might be tempted to increase the weight but usually what happens is that people start to have bad form, rock forward, and possibly strain their back. Start by just standing up and take it from there. Be smart and don't sacrifice time off the water due to preventable injury.

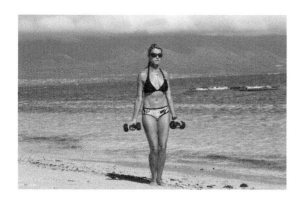 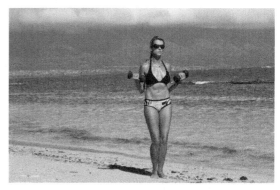

As in Progressions 1 and 2, you can do regular and hammer curls with 2 arms or alternating. I mix it up myself.

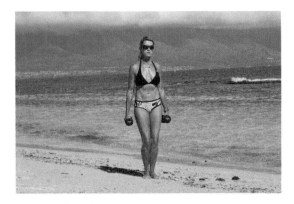 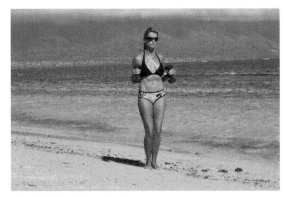

I suggest that you stand with your feet shoulder width apart, knees slightly bent and maintaining excellent posture throughout your set. If you can't do this then stay seated.

Now you can go from two legs to one. It's kind of fun and keeps your interest. Remember this is a strength exercise first. So if you're not having great balance here, keep it to two legs firmly on the ground.

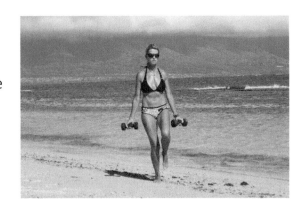

PROGRESSION 3

If you're up for some fun and want to keep your guns firing like canons, step up onto the BOSU. Your legs will get a nice firing as well, as will your core muscles. Again, don't go too heavy with the weights and remember that your focus is on your biceps.

With the BOSU dome up, step up with two feet, not too wide, and bring your dumbbells with you. Always keep your knees slightly bent, and everything else you know the same as in Progression 1. It's a lot of fun and you should keep things moving smoothly without bouncing too much.

Perform your regular, hammer curls with two arms or alternating. I do not recommend doing this on one leg. Always stand on two for your safety and success.

PROGRESSION 4

Now you can bring out the half foam roller or the Gigante Flo Cushion and Indo Board of choice and really mix up the fun.

I'd start with the half foam roller with one foot. Then two feet placed on half foam roller in a horizontal fashion. Lastly, you can attempt a two leg or one leg challenge on top of the Gigante Flo Cushion, nubby side up with board placed on it. Refer to photos below. I'm not smiling because these are frigg'n hard and it was hot. Good luck!

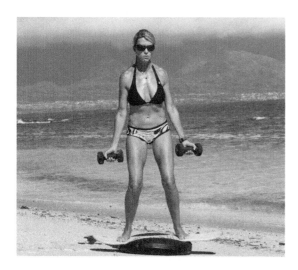 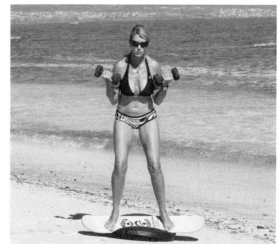

Exercise 2:
BASIC CURLS RESISTANCE TUBING

It's good to have choices and challenge the same muscles with different equipment. By using the resistance tubing you're creating a different kind of load and challenge. Go easy on this as we don't want to transfer the effort to the forearm—known as forearm pump.

SUGGESTED TRAINING EQUIPMENT
Resistance tubing, Indo Board of choice if needed

SUGGESTED REPS/SETS
12-20, 1-2 sets

MOVEMENT TEMPO/SPEED
Controlled with good form

PROGRESSION VARIABLES
Increase tube gauge, 2-1 leg, increase second hold time for each rep

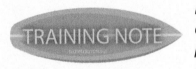

Because I often train at the beach and am barefoot, I don't want to step directly on the tubing as it would really pinch and hurt. I use the Indo Board to help as my base. It works great. You can also use this in your home.

Take a medium gauge resistance tube and lay the tubing on the ground. With a hand in each handle, step to the center of the tubing. Really bend the knees and put into practice your shoulder retraction.

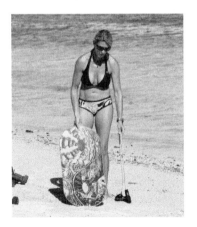
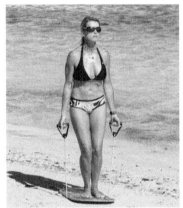
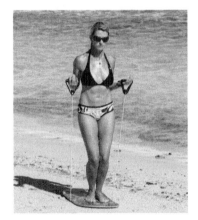

Rise up slightly, chest out, and pull the tubing up towards you like a dumbbell curl. I suggest you only perform as a two arm exercise and don't grab the handles too tight. You will fatigue quicker than you think.

Keep the elbows close to your rib cage and don't allow them to fly up and away. Good job.

Now here is the same exercise on one leg:

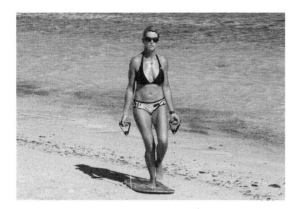 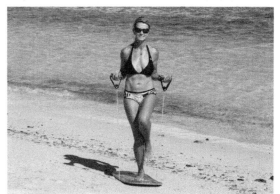

TRICEPS

The triceps, plural, technically called the triceps brachii for the Latin meaning "three headed arm muscle" are often misunderstood and neglected when it comes to improving stand up paddling performance.

The triceps help you get back up on your board when you fall off. They also help stabilize your shoulder blades and help you extend your elbow for those powerful strokes forward and for those strokes when you're just warming up. They are also critical when bringing your arm back toward your body to begin the next stroke.

When these muscles are weak and undertrained your entire SUP experience is hindered and unbalanced.

You've already been giving your triceps some love while you were training the chest. Now the focus is strictly on them.

SUGGESTED TRAINING EQUIPMENT
Dumbbells 5-10 pounds, TRX Rip Trainer, weight bench or chair, resistance tubing

SUGGESTED REPS/SETS
12-20, 1-2 sets

MOVEMENT TEMPO/SPEED
Controlled with good form,1-3 second hold

PROGRESSION VARIABLES
2-1 arm, add weight accordingly, standing or seated

Exercise 1:
SIMPLE 1-2 ARM TRICEP KICKBACKS, STANDING OR SEATED

PROGRESSION 1

This is your basic old-school tricep exercise that is really simple and effective. I'd start with one arm to get the basics down then you can work your way up to two.

With one dumbbell in your right hand, stand in a staggered stance with the left leg forward and the left arm supported on your thigh. Bend over at the hip, keeping your back straight and your head and neck neutral, looking down at ground. With your elbow bent—now it's near your waist—keep it tucked in close to your body at the same level as your back. (See photo below.) Press back and up towards ceiling to straighten arm. Hold 1-2 seconds and return arm to start at side.

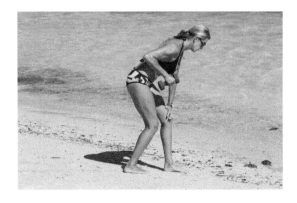 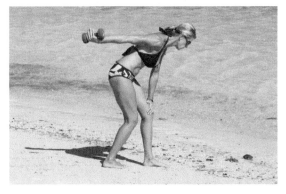

PROGRESSION 2

If you'd like to do two arms at once I recommend using lighter weights. You can assume the same stance and it doesn't matter which leg you put forward as long as your head is neutral.

To assure good form, gently squeeze shoulder blades to help stabilize your body throughout the movement. You want to keep your elbows pinned at your rib cage. Look down and press back. Increase the intensity by adding a second hold. Don't sacrifice good form for heavier weights. Maintain a steady and smooth set.

PROGRESSION 3

You can also perform the two arm progression sitting down in a chair or on a weight bench. I like to sit on my bench so I can give full attention to the muscle. With two feet on the floor and together, bend over at the hip, retract your shoulder blades and assume a nice straight line from head to lower back and look down at the ground. Don't allow your head to jut forward.

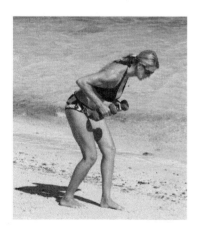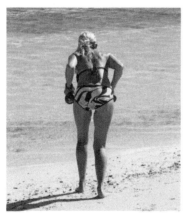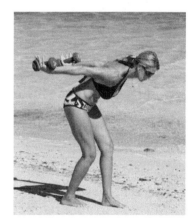

Press back or kick back the dumbbells together behind you with a breath out. Hold if you like to add some extra juice to the tricep muscles.

Exercise 2:
TRX RIP TRAINER OVERHEAD PRESSES

This one takes some practice and requires you to really be the stabilizing force for smooth execution. You become a tower of power. You will be working the triceps but you'll also notice and feel your shoulders and back assisting you.

Safety is number one on this to take note.

SUGGESTED TRAINING EQUIPMENT
TRX Rip Trainer, heavy cord

SUGGESTED REPS/SETS
15-20, 1-2 sets

MOVEMENT TEMPO/SPEED
Controlled with good form,1-3 second hold

PROGRESSION VARIABLES
1-3 second holds, changing tempo and speed of movement

Just as you did in the back and chest exercises with the Rip Trainer, secure the cord around a pole or use the door jam accessory and place at shoulder height. This is higher than you have placed it before. You may need to make small adjustments as you go.

Step inside the cord and Rip Trainer. Secure the safety loop to your hand and grab the middle part of bar on each end. Raise the bar with your hands above your head, slightly behind your head, elbows bent and with your eyes looking forward.

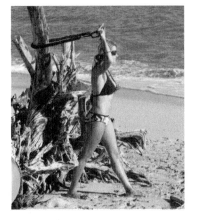 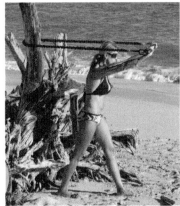

Assume a staggered stance to best stabilize you. You may lean slightly forward. You'll then press the bar forward and let the elbows almost lock, while breathing out. Here's where the triceps feel it. It may take a few reps to get a smooth rhythm.

You can adjust the tension if necessary and experiment with a 1-3 second hold. It's tricky but you'll get it with practice.

Exercise 3:
TUBE PRESS DOWNS

This is one of the simpler ones that I do all the time and, wow, do they ever make my triceps strong. It does require similar prep as the Standing Back Tube Presses but they're so worth the quick set up.

I love it when I see my clients' triceps wink back at me.

SUGGESTED TRAINING EQUIPMENT
Resistance tubing

SUGGESTED REPS/SETS
15-20, 1-2 sets

MOVEMENT TEMPO/SPEED
Controlled with good form,1-3 second hold

PROGRESSION VARIABLES
1-3 second holds, changing tempo and speed of movement, adjust tension or tubing gauge, or 2-1 legs

---

This time the tubing gets secured about 2-3 feet above your head. You can use a hook of some sort or use the door jam accessory, but make sure whatever you use is super solid.

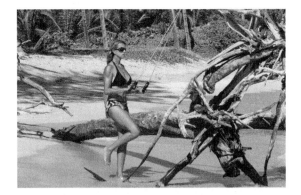

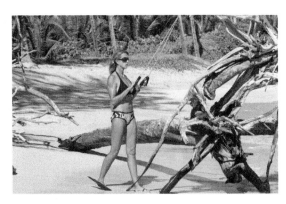

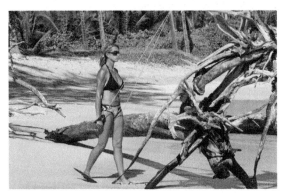

Grab a handle in each hand and face the hook or door in a staggered stance. Step back about a foot. Do your pelvic tilt forward, pull your shoulders back, and secure your shoulder blades in retraction. All of this assures an excellent outcome.

Your eyes are gazing forward, neck relaxed, and elbows are tight to your body. Press down the tubing to slightly past your thighs.

Don't let your shoulders rise up to your ears or let your elbows fly up. Press and repeat. Adjust tension as needed and experiment with the second hold.

Exercise 4:
BENCH DIPS

Again, another old-school favorite that is quite challenging as you have to use your own body weight. If you are not able to do push ups too well you may want to pass on this one.

As you build your strength you can shift the emphasis on how much work your triceps actually do. Get some help from your legs in the beginning. You can do this by placing your feet, at first, about shoulder-width apart. Then gradually bring your feet closer together. Ultimately you can switch between each leg and then repeat with feet on the BOSU to decrease your stability.

SUGGESTED TRAINING EQUIPMENT
Sturdy bench, sturdy downed tree

SUGGESTED REPS/SETS
12-20, 1-2 sets

MOVEMENT TEMPO/SPEED
Controlled with good form, 1-3 second hold

PROGRESSION VARIABLES
2-1 leg, flat feet to heels to BOSU

PROGRESSION 1

Sit in the middle of the bench or on the tree with knees bent at 90 degrees. Place your hands close to your thighs on the bench and your feet in front of you. Walk both feet forward just a bit so that your butt is off the bench and you're supporting your upper body securely. Lower yourself down towards ground and then push yourself back up. Repeat.

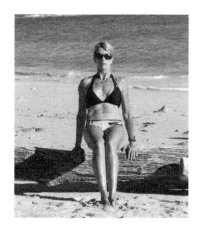
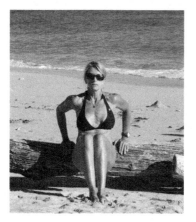
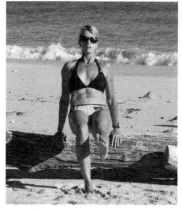

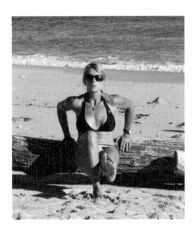 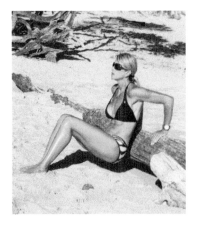 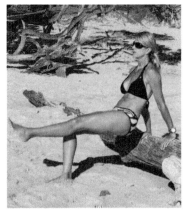

To increase this challenge, bring your feet close together. Then, to add one more strength component, lift one leg straight out and give that a try. This last move is very challenging.

PROGRESSION 2

Assume same position as above and, this time, extend your legs with your weight resting on your heels versus flat feet. As simple as this change is, this is really difficult and will put you a little closer to the ground. You'll quickly find out if your shoulders are weak. Lower yourself down the ground but be sure you can come back up!

For the ultimate challenge, place your heels on the BOSU then attempt the exercise on one leg:

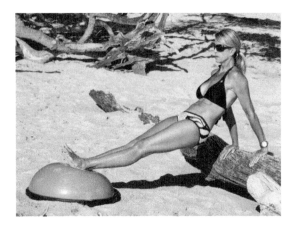 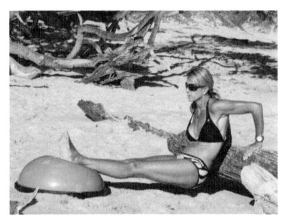

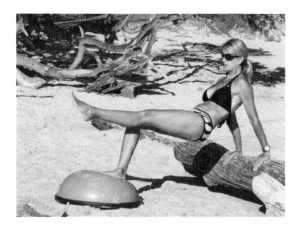 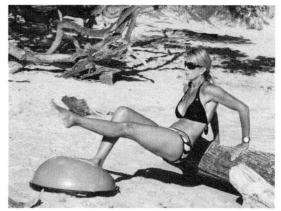

Now that you've learned and completed these exercises, let me know and I'll call the contractor to widen the door for you, or at least carry your board for you at the next race as your reward.

You must feel great and powerful right now. I'm sure you're able to paddle over tall waves in a few strokes while passing your competitors with a big smile and grace! They may not see you because your biceps shadow is blocking the light of the sun.

All fun aside, great job!

Coming up next in Chapter 5, you'll begin your training to improve leg strength to connect your core, your balance, and your upper body strength into one fine paddling machine.

CHAPTER 5
Stronger Legs Equal Huge Gains in SUP Performance

- How leg strength improves your stand up paddling.
- The importance of breaking down each point of leg strength for SUP.
- Making the transition to waves.
- Learning to dance to catch downwind glides.
- Improving total leg endurance for long distance paddling.
- Strength and endurance building exercises for your legs.

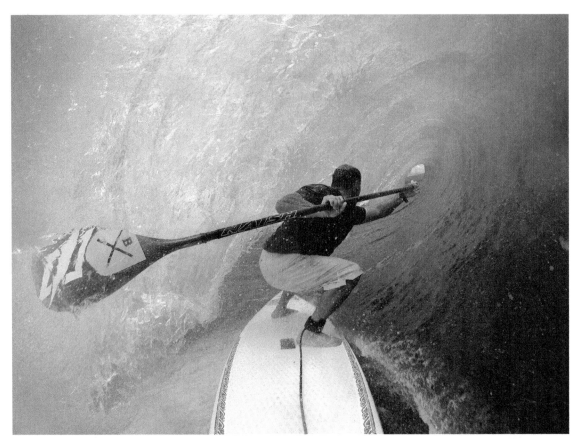

Loch Eggers Photo by Darrell Wong

From beginners to professional paddlers, everyone can benefit from having strong legs. In this chapter I'll show you how to maximize your leg strength and endurance so you can enjoy paddling longer, reduce the likelihood of being injured, push your limits, and improve your overall stand up paddling performance.

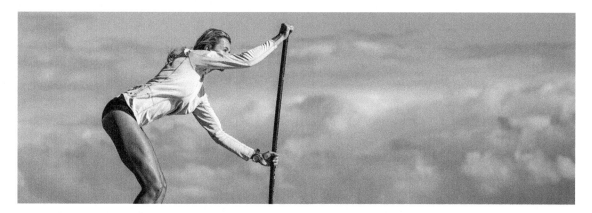

Training your legs to be stronger for SUP will help you react quickly to changing conditions such as side chop or swell and will increase your muscle endurance for channel crossings and distance races. Strong paddling legs will also allow you to deliver more power from the hips to your feet so that you can propel your board faster at the start of race.

Most people rely only on the larger muscles of the legs and generally think of their legs as one unit in stand up paddling. If you can start thinking of each leg as acting independently as well as together, you can literally start shifting more power to the board.

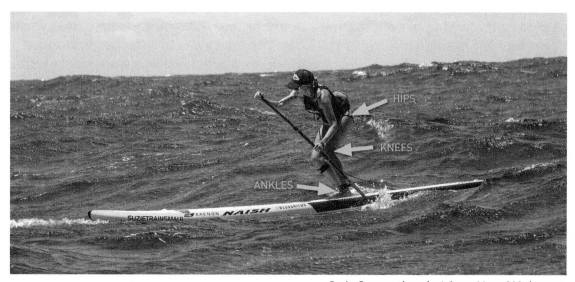

Suzie Cooney photo by Johann Meya 808photome

Next you can learn to recognize how each joint of the leg, including the hip, knee, and ankle joints, play important roles in your success and performance. And, finally, you can zero in and focus on the tiny, finer muscles supporting each joint—including the tendons and ligaments. That is when your skills will go from good to *great*.

Here's an example of the points I mention above. Let's say you're at a local SUP race on the lake. The morning is calm and the course has three buoy turns. Sounds simple to me. Your division has around 30 people and your start time is later in morning when you know the wind will come up.

You line up and your heart is pounding out of your chest as you wait for the horn. You thrust up to your feet (glutes and thighs), you take that first dig in (feet and ankles stabilize you), you push hard to thrust forward, and you get into the top 5 fast (hips and knees). Then a huge gust of wind comes across the lake out of nowhere at the first turn. There's water chop from all of the other paddlers coming in all directions and it's like paddling in chunky soup. You've practiced this turn a hundred times, but wait—someone has just tapped the tail of your board, hard, and there is no way you are going down.

Every ounce of you wants to stay on the board in that turn, even with Ram Rod Richie or Rhonda behind you. Who you gonna call? SUP Bouncers or SUPBusters?

No, you're calling on all of your brain and ALL the muscles of your feet, ankles, knees, hips, and your brain to keep you upright. The tiny muscles are fighting together with the large muscles to help you around that first turn. THIS IS WAR.

All kidding aside, I hope this gives you a better picture that you can relate to as you begin your leg strength training in this book. The take away here is the importance of excelling in your stand up paddling performance with both legs working in unison together and independently of each other.

TRANSITIONING TO WAVES

Now not all of you can get inside the barrels on your first spin out like our Loch Eggers here. But the reason I selected this photo was to show how much rail pressure Loch is creating. He's pressing his right rear foot literally into the face of wave to help hold him down the line for speed and depth.

You can see every fine muscle of the outer part of his calves firing to get that firm plant of his left (forward) foot. This also helps him to steer his board.

He didn't learn this overnight and, yes, he does paddle at JAWS and some of our other huge outer reefs, but he does so with strength and lots of big wave knowledge.

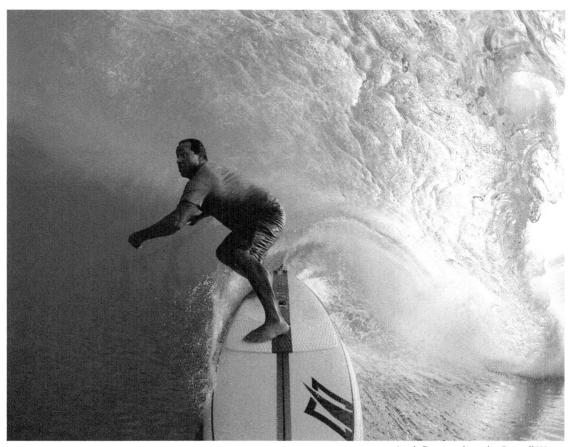

Loch Eggers photo by Darrell Wong

I get so many emails from people who ask me, "How should I be training and what can I do to make myself a better and stronger paddle surfer?"

When you're making the transition from flat water to wave paddling, it's all about footwork and reading the water. You'll want to learn all you can about how to time the waves. It's pretty awesome when you can train your body to connect to your brain's intention and have it all right there at the end of your paddle and under your feet.

I'd like to stop here for one very important message to all of you who are thinking of getting into SUP paddle surfing. Please learn all you can about wave safety and wave etiquette BEFORE you venture out, even if it's in 1-2 feet ankle biters.

You can have a really, really, awesome day in the waves or a really, really, bad day. You could cause harm to someone else and/or yourself because you didn't know the "right of way," were not in control of your gear, were in over your head, or even, the worst case scenario, all of the above.

Always wear a leash and check the string that attaches to the board because that ultimately attaches to the leash to the board. Your board can become a rocket and a fast moving torpedo into someone's back or in path of another paddler or surfer. Check your leash for damage and integrity and replace as often as possible, as leashes get stretched out and can weaken over time.

Learn how to control your board in small and big surf. You will earn great respect quickly if you can manage your gear and yourself and keep everyone, including yourself, safe. When things get ugly on a bad wipeout or small wipeout, and you lose your paddle, ALWAYS GO TO YOUR BOARD FIRST. That is your life line and flotation device. On bigger waves, some of us wear impact vests that help one "pop up" a bit more quickly in case of extreme hold downs. It can, literally, get really heavy really quickly.

Our passion for SUP is real and if you want to be more accepted and treated well with respect from other fellow surfing friends, please study and learn to be a paddle surfing ambassador not a hazard. This also goes for being able to "give a lot and take a few." Being a SUP star doesn't mean you get to be a wave hog.

If you'd like to learn more about SUP wave etiquette and safety, check out my FREE, 3 part video called *SUP Pro Talk with Suzie Cooney Wave Safety and Etiquette, Gear Talk and more*, with special guests Jeremy Riggs and Clay Everline, M.D. co author and surfer of the booked called Surf Survival, The Surfer's Health Handbook. Check out the model.

In Chapter 3 I introduced you to balance training. The exercises I suggested play a huge role in your leg strength training as well. As you start progressing your paddle surf skills, you should revisit those often, if not every time you train, in order to keep your legs in shape for paddle surfing.

Also included in that chapter was an exercise to help you make your first step in transitioning from normal stance to surf stance. That kind of leg strength is also a confidence-building factor geared toward getting you to the point where you feel like you can go for it! If you have the leg strength you'll have the confidence.

Your footwork will simply take practice, as will your ability to automatically place your feet in the right position on the board to catch the wave. If you have good to great leg strength that will help you all the more to successfully catch small to big waves.

As you become *really* good on the waves, you'll be able to distinguish just how much more leg strength you'll need to hold the rail on the face of wave to stay high or to carve a nice bottom turn—all of which require extra leg strength.

In this photo you can really see how Loch Eggers' calf muscles are firing as he braces his paddle against the wave for extra leverage. Very cool and impressive.

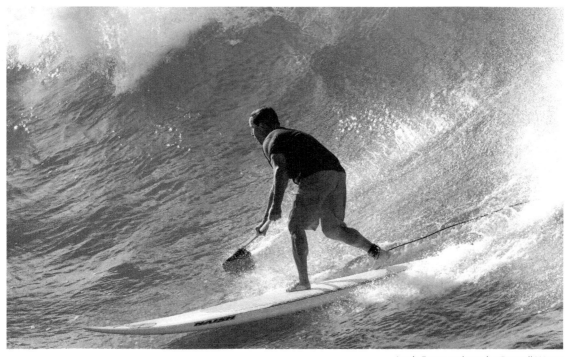

Loch Eggers photo by Darrell Wong

For the more advanced wave paddlers who may be going a bit deeper and bigger this season, rail pressure and back leg strength are super important. Once you make the drop you'll need leg strength as you begin to build speed. Then, as you're shooting across the wave, you might do a quick push back up the face for a nice cut back and then pump and compress again to regain your momentum. If the wave is especially long and clean you'll certainly have time to do this. If your legs are weak and undertrained, you might get one decent bottom turn and then have to kick out.

So, from beginner wave SUP chargers to the pros, everyone wins with strong legs for wave paddling.

THE ART OF THE DOWNWIND DANCE

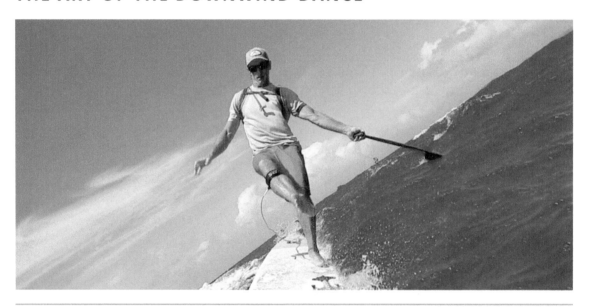

Jeremy Riggs shows off his signature dance moves! May I please have this dance Jeremy?

I love to downwind paddle and catch bumps and glides; I think of it as kind of a dance. What I mean by that is that I use footwork, balance, and leg strength to give me the confidence to step— sometimes even taking a double step in one movement—all the way back so I'm over the fin of a 14 or 16 foot or even an 18 foot board to catch a glide.

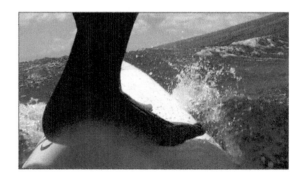

How to Increase Your Stand Up Paddling Performance

One of the most amazing pairs of light feet and strong legs (Jill Riggs, wife to Jeremy Riggs, don't take this the wrong way please) are attached to one of the legends around here, my good friend and coach, Jeremy Riggs. I'm just saying he can dance on the *narrowest* of downwind boards and makes it look so easy.

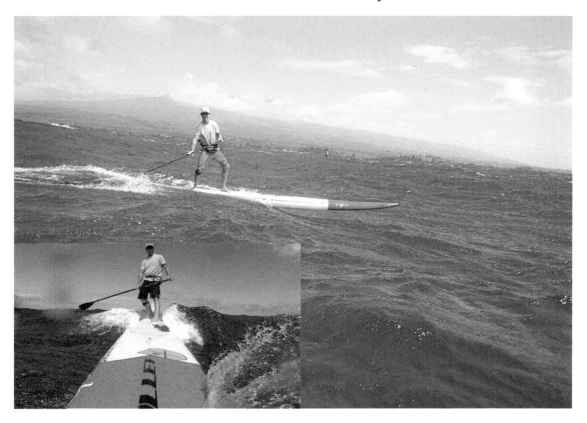

Jeremy Riggs

Jeremy is also my coach for downwinding and THE downwind expert on Maui. He's relaxed and light on his feet but you can be sure he's powerful in his upper body as well. The pros like Jeremy just make it look easy. Take note of the movement of his entire body. He's totally relaxed: chest open, back towards the fin—letting the board find the best line. Once that glide commences he will walk back toward the middle of the board, catch the next bump and step back again.

Connor Baxter is another one who's got some fancy moves. Those moves are more than just something pretty to look at. What the ability to dance around the board equates to is incredible efficiency so you can save energy and make catching all the bumps, big or small, worthwhile.

When you've mastered the footwork techniques, and the winds are light, being agile and light on your feet can put you many board lengths ahead. Just wait until you combine that with powerful legs that help you thrust your hips and board forward.

I always tell people if you can't dance you won't catch bumps and glides. Peeps, you've gotta have rhythm. You need to be smooth and graceful and put a little finesse into your footwork before your blade even touches the water. Because you're "surfing" most of the time, you'll be burning out the fine muscles AND the larger muscles of your legs for miles.

When you get into downwind paddling, having leg strength will also help you position your weight and hold a hard line in challenging conditions, such as big, windy swells. Here's JR again, holding this board on the face of a big downwind wave and swell!

At times I've felt my thigh muscles burning when I've had to hold down the rail on one side of my downwind board to help me paddle into the wind on heavy days. When this happens, my confidence soars, and I'm able to keep up with other strong paddlers; it feels great.

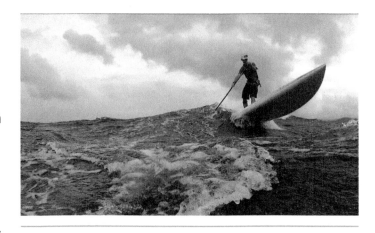

Jeremy Riggs

Living on Maui we are so lucky to have our famous 10-mile downwind magic carpet ride, known as the Maliko run. On the very best days you literally surf 9 of those miles, and I sure feel it in my legs! It's freaking amazing.

I'll go into a little more detail on footwork when we talk about cardio strength for downwind paddling in Chapter 6.

GOING THE DISTANCE WITH YOUR LEGS IN STAND UP PADDLING

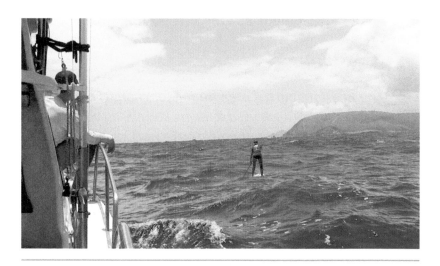

Suzie Cooney paddling M20 2104 as Coach Jeremy Riggs looks on.

As I write this book I'm currently training a client from Bermuda to paddle around the entire island, a distance of approximately 45 miles. I've written a progressive, distance and training plan to help him build up his total leg and body endurance.

He recently reported back on his first 25 miler and was happy to say that he felt good. He thought his feet would fall asleep (a common occurrence for some), but they did not. He did share that his ankles were sore and tired.

Looking back to my training for the M20, to prepare for that distance and endurance I'd often do "double" 10 mile Malikos, or 20 miles, back to back. Although I had a relay partner for that race I needed to uncover my weak points in the legs. I needed to see how my legs withstood standing on the board for long periods of time.

This was not easy. Because of serious leg injuries in 2009 my circulation near my ankles is quite challenged. There was no other way to prepare. I just had to paddle. When I actually did the crossing, I was well prepared. My ankles did exhibit some fatigue but it wasn't anything I couldn't handle.

There are many things to consider when training for channel crossings or for distance paddling. Besides having a strong mental game, which I talk about more in Chapter 7, you really have to put some miles on your legs to prepare them. There's no magic number of miles you need to complete, as everyone is different.

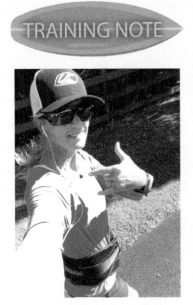

An important part of preparation for channel crossings or distance is to get used to being literally on your feet for long periods of time. You're working hard and moving back and forth from normal stance to surf stance constantly, as well, especially in the channels off Maui.

By walking with a weight belt, you can load your legs with up to 10lbs of more force production which will help build this endurance. In this photo I'm preparing for the M2M or Maui to Molokai, 27 miles of standing and surfing in open-ocean.

Do not jog or run with weight belt.

Some people experiment with compression pants and some actually wear supportive booties with custom orthotic inserts. What it comes down to is how your legs maintain overall total endurance with each mile.

Your training approach should combine cardio, balance, and a combination of training exercises for the entire leg complex of muscles. I also suggest you give yourself plenty of time to prepare before an event or before you set a goal to train accordingly and log your miles. Make note of how your legs feel per five miles, 10 miles, and at each additional five mile increment. More on this in Chapter 8.

There are many benefits to training your legs for stand up paddling so check out this chapter to learn more.

LEGS

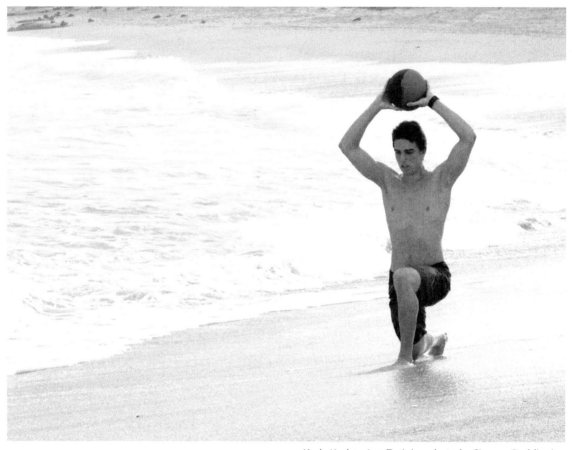

Kody Kerbox Leg Training photo by Simone Reddingius

Exercise 1:
STANDARD LEG SQUATS & CHALLENGING PROGRESSIONS

You know how awesome it feels when you stick a nice pivot turn around a buoy, or nail a sweet wave, or catch a glide and ride it like an ocean cowboy (or cowgirl) with a big smile and grin. No doubt your legs stoked your stroke and stroked your stoke! Say that three times fast. In any and all of those paddling experiences your hips, quad muscles, hamstrings, calves, knees and shins, were working overtime. Insert a "woot woot" here.

I'm starting with this exercise first because it's simple and straightforward. However, I can make this ultra challenging so your legs will shake like Jell-O. That's *my* goal. I have **A LOT** of special progressions that you can work towards so pace yourself. Your legs will reward you with more adventures on the water.

SUGGESTED TRAINING EQUIPMENT

5-15 pound dumbbells, half foam roller, 10-20 pound kettlebell, BOSU, stability ball, Indo Board of choice, 24" Gigante Flo Cushion, 8-10 pound medicine ball, full length mirror

SUGGESTED REPS/SETS

12-15, 1-2 sets

MOVEMENT TEMPO/SPEED

Controlled with 1-3 second holds

PROGRESSION VARIABLES

Floor to BOSU, to Indo Board of choice to 24" Gigante Flo Cushion, no weights to weights, 2-1 leg weights above shoulder or at knee level

PROGRESSION 1

The standard squat is a good place to start your leg training to increase your base of strength for stand up paddling. From here I'll increase your challenge to include the finer muscles that support the larger muscles such as your quads, hamstring and glutes.

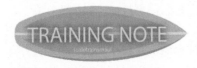 *Remember to always include also the balance exercises from Chapter 3 as those are also helping improve your leg strength.*

Proper form for squats is important so if you haven't used one already, this is the best time to perform in front of a full length mirror to watch for any points of compensation. I will help you learn how to cue and observe your movements and range of motion.

Begin with your feet shoulder width apart, toes pointing straight. Take your hands and simply gently hold or clasp them together at chest level in front of your body. Now, as you lower yourself by bending your knees, maintain good posture and be sure your heels don't cave in or lift off the ground. Also try and keep your knees tracking over your second toe throughout the entire motion of your squat.

Should your knees buckle inward or outward you may need to adjust your width of feet and/or maybe not go down as deep. (This is a possible indication that your muscles are out of balance—some are over active and/or under active. So please be mindful during these exercises. It's not a bad thing, just something you should be aware of.) Do not bend your knees past 90 degrees. As you rise back up to the start position, please do not fully lock your knees. Repeat and watch your form.

PROGRESSION 2

Add Weights

Most people start with 8 pounds and go up from there. There are two positions to hold the dumbbells; each offers a difference load force to the legs.

Position 1: Simply hold at your side just near the thigh. As you lower yourself down for the squat, keep your arms straight, maintain great posture, and return to start position. Try and feel the emphasis from the ground, to the heel up to your butt. Repeat.

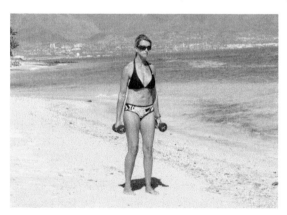
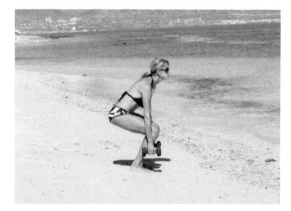

Position 2: Now take each dumbbell and gently rest one end on the top of your shoulder. Begin your squat and feel the load above your legs. It's a different shift of strength. You will definitely feel this.

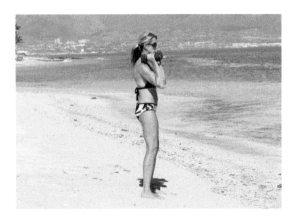 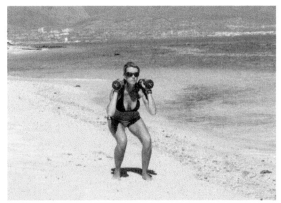

You can mix up this variation between sets and you can apply to all of the exercises for legs moving forward.

PROGRESSION 3

Single Leg Pistol Squats

Okay, let's just get these done. All I know is that these are hard and I sincerely feel that this exercise is for the very, very conditioned and advanced paddlers. As always, common sense rules. Don't get discouraged! You will achieve success and the results are rock hard legs. Commit and your body will reward you.

Prerequisites: *To be able to perform at least 40 good quality two-legged squats with excellent form. Additionally be able to squat past 90 degrees without compensation or discomfort or loss of stability. Finally, to be injury free and have very good flexibility at the hip, knee and ankle.*

Your form for this must be spot on. The good news is that because these are so intense you can perform fewer due the high quality demand in nature. It's easier to complete this exercise while wearing training shoes.

As with the two-legged squat, it is best to practice good posture and track your knee over your second long toe. Because I am not wearing shoes, in the photos for this exercise I've placed the Indo Board underneath me to add to stability.

Start by extending both arms in front of you as you stand on one leg. Lower yourself into your first pistol squat and have your foot go out in front of you. Keep focused, foot flat on the ground. There is a chance you could fall on your butt a couple of times, and you may discover one leg to be stronger than the other, but keep at it.

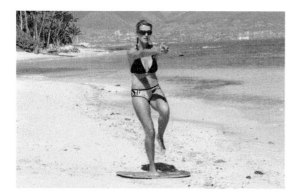 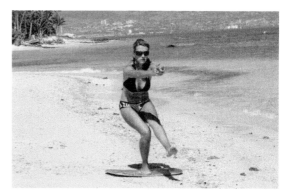

As you push back up to start you'll REALLY feel your glute or butt muscles fire. This is good. I'd do about 5-10 reps on each leg. You may progress to the half foam roller if you choose or hold a medicine ball or dumbbell out in front of you.

Only go down as far as you can manage solid form.

PROGRESSION 4

Wall Squat With Stability Ball 2-1 Leg

This one is great for anyone who had trouble with the standard squat variables, but offers its own different levels of intensity. Place the stability ball behind you in the small of your back. Spread feet shoulder width apart and just forward of knees. Keep knees slightly bent.

Next, with your hands in front of you and off your body, lower hips toward the floor until they reach knee height. At that point stop and return to starting position without allowing your knees to lock, then repeat. I'd be very careful not to go past 90 degrees.

You can also experiment by moving feet a bit closer together, and/or out a bit and then move feet very close together. That is really challenging!

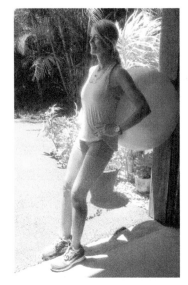

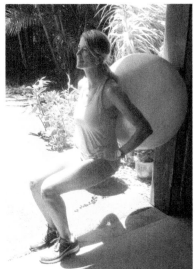

You can add weights too, as you did above in the same two positions—hold at your side and on top of your shoulder. You'll REALLY feel this so maybe split up your sets and try different positions.

The key is not to rely on wall or ball too much while performing these and remember to always keep a slight bend of the knee as you complete each rep.

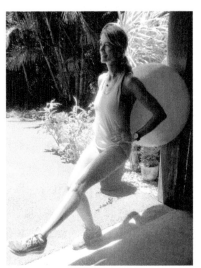

Finally, if you're really digging these, attempt all the above on one leg. I highly suggest you work up to this level slowly and maybe attempt five on each leg. Be sure that your knee is tracking nicely in alignment with second long toe and do not go too deep in your squat.

PROGRESSION 4

Squat on BOSU

This is a blast as long as you're using good form with excellent posture. If the BOSU is inflated to its max it will be easier. If it's inflated with less air it's quite a bit more challenging. I also suggest that you perform this one in front of your full- length mirror for self-cuing.

With the BOSU dome side up step up with your two feet on top of BOSU. Your feet will be a bit less than shoulder width apart. If they are too wide, your form will be sloppy. Starting as you would a regular squat, gently clasp your hands in front of you, and begin your squat. Do not let your legs go past a 90 degree bend. As you rise back up to the start position it's important not to lock your knees. Keep them softly bent.

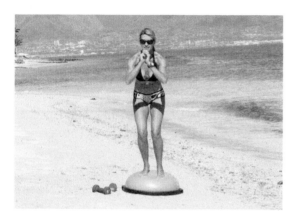 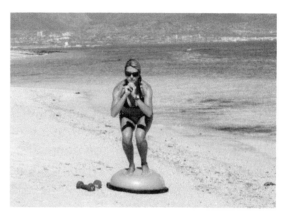

You can also progress this exercise with weights, holding at your side or on top of the shoulders. To add a little extra thunder to your thighs, hold each squat for 2-3 seconds.

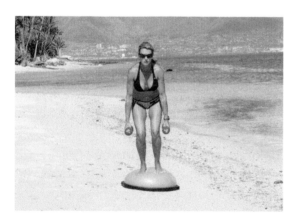 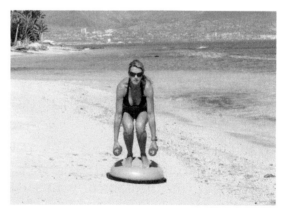

When you step off, let me know which flavor JELL-O you are! Good job.

PROGRESSION 5

This one really calls for the best form as possible. (Be careful, this could cause you to laugh hysterically at yourself.) **Grab your half foam roller** and place in front of you horizontally.

Step up with two feet and immediately bend your knees. If you lock them at any time, you could end up "rolling down the windows." (Flailing your arms around.) It's just like paddling when you're learning. If you stand upright too fast and lock the knees you're guaranteed to do the Nestea® plunge.

Bring your arms straight out in front of you and attempt your first squat. The mirror really helps, so laser focus on those knees tracking over your second long toe as best as possible. Don't go too deep. The key is to lean forward like you would down a wave. This is a tricky one. *(You will notice in photo, because I was at the beach, I placed a half foam roller on top of Indo Board Kick Tail for stability. Works great.)*

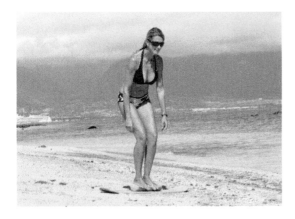 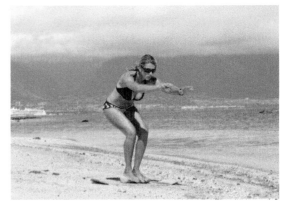

To add to the intensity but also as a counter balance, grab a medicine ball or one dumbbell and hold it in both hands while you complete your squat. As you squat you can push the medicine ball out and in, out and then in. Keep breathing and keep practicing.

PROGRESSION 6

Squat on Indo Board of Choice & Gigante Flo Cushion

Now that you're the squat king or queen, let's have some extra fun and add some flavors to your JELL-O pack variety.

As you paddle, there really is no sweet spot on your board. You're always moving— as is the water underneath you. So the more we mimic that notion and motion the better paddler you'll become and that's why we're here.

Some people have a love/hate relationship with this exercise so I'll share the love with you first then you can decide. Our goals are the same: burn out all the leg muscles to fatigue so we can build our overall leg endurance.

Place the Gigante Flo Cushion nubby side up and center your board on top and horizontally. (Less inflation of the cushion is more difficult vs. inflation at 50%) See photo. Depending upon your level of comfort and experience on the gear, adjust the width of your feet accordingly. Keep in mind, too wide and your body mechanics won't be that great. Too close and the exercise then becomes too much of a balance focus.

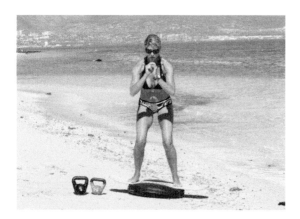 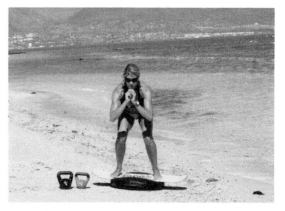

Find your ideal foot width so you can manage a proper squat and begin your first squat. Keep a slight lean forward and give it your best. Because there is so much action with the cushion versus the BOSU take your time and don't rush. Once you've completed a full set you can add weight in the two positions you've learned.

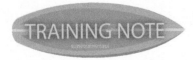

If you selected the Indo Board Pro Kicktail I highly suggest you start with lighter weights since this is a narrower board.

You can also try this: Grab a kettle bell, say 10-15 pounds, and, with two hands, you can load your squat as you would with two dumbbells. To add total earthquake chaos and another challenging variable, hold that squat for 2-3 seconds. This will quickly fatigue you. I always say, "Shake and bake, just shake and bake."

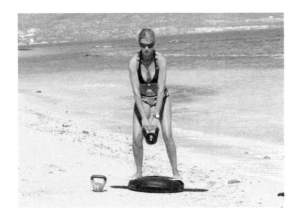 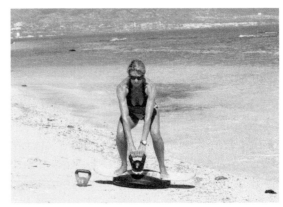

Finally, I've saved the best progression for last. With the same kettle bell raise it above your shoulder and rest it on the bicep and perform your squat. Here, like the other dumbbell position variables, this will cause yet another earthquake. Your own tremor will depend on your leg strength, balance and endurance. It's an awesome challenge.

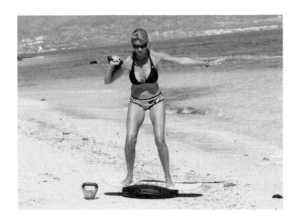 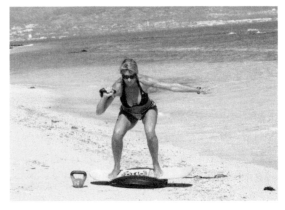

Exercise 2:
TWO LEG HAMSTRING CURLS ON STABILITY BALL

I'll be honest I often get a few grumbles on this one, but once you get it you'll love the challenge. The hamstring muscles are important to SUP because they're crucial strength stabilizers you use when making weight shifts on the water. The hamstring muscles additionally assist you in securely planting your back leg for carving on a wave or during foot transitions from your normal stance to a surfing downwind stance, as shown in my photo below.

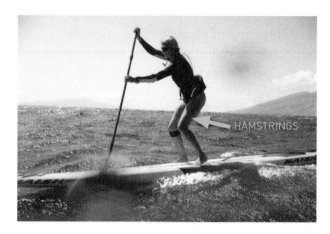

This exercise will help strengthen the back of your legs so that your kneecap functions properly and tracks accordingly, along with the tendons to keep it stable throughout your normal and/or intense paddling sessions. If your hamstring muscles are strong they will also assist your glutes in protecting your lower back for long distance races and channel crossings.

SUGGESTED TRAINING EQUIPMENT
Stability ball, floor mat

SUGGESTED REPS/SETS
12-15, 1-2 sets

MOVEMENT TEMPO/SPEED
Controlled with 1-2 second holds

PROGRESSION VARIABLES
2-1 leg

PROGRESSION 1

Place mat on the floor. Sit at the edge of the mat with stability ball. Lay back with entire back, shoulders and neck on the mat with your arms at your side. Bend your knees at 90 degrees and place your heels a top of the stability ball.

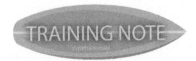 This is best performed with shoes and with a firm stability ball.

Lift your hips up off the mat and curl your heels toward your glutes by bending your knees. Slowly return to the start position while maintaining the level of your hips throughout the entire exercise. Do not allow the feet to externally rotate while flexing the knees. (Keep toes pointing straight up.)

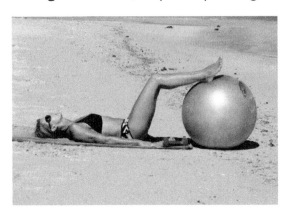 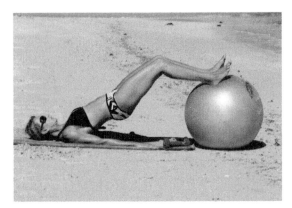

Do not allow your hips to drop while flexing the knees. If your hips continue to drop descend the progression by performing the hip extension only.

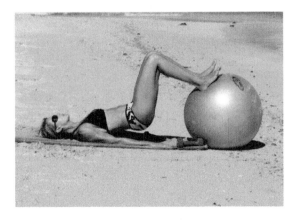

At first you might be a little wobbly but keep at it. Once you get a few sets completed you'll get the hang of it. It's important you don't cramp up during the exercise. You will also feel your calf muscles fire at this time and that is normal.

PROGRESSION 2

Once you've got those harp cords used to the tension and you've avoided cramping up, you may attempt to perform five or more reps with one leg. You must have complete control of the stability ball at all times throughout the entire set.

As in Progression 1, start with both heels on top of the stability ball and lift your hips up towards the ceiling. Carefully lift one leg off the ball and curl the ball towards your butt. This can be very intense and if you didn't cramp before, you might now.

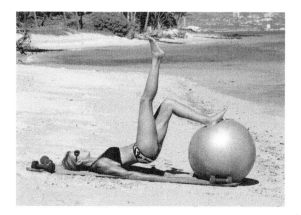 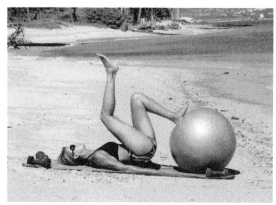

Don't allow the lifted leg to meander about. Just bend the knee and keep it in close to your body. Go easy. These are not pretty but they are good for your legs.

Exercise 3:
STEP/BOX STEP UP

Although you may be eager to have legs and buns of carbon, good things take time. So as you go back and fine-tune your stroke, we're going back to a simple old-school leg strength exercise.

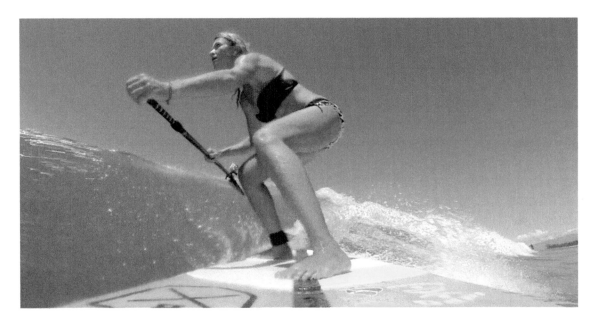

If you want to catch more waves this exercise is vital to your success. Your legs need to be SOLID and strong to maximize each ride down the line. You need your glutes, hamstring muscles and quads to act as one so you can control the board, compress back up and do it again and again.

The act of stepping up on a box tones and strengthens your legs, period. It sounds simple enough and it is. Simple is good. The more challenging exercises are waiting for you below after you perform this well.

I have an adjustable step up box and a tall, fixed wooden box. Just be sure it's sturdy and can handle your weight. Shoes are suggested.

SUGGESTED TRAINING EQUIPMENT
5-15 pound dumbbells, sturdy box or step 6 inches to 36 inches tall, full length mirror

SUGGESTED REPS/SETS
12-15, 1-2 sets

MOVEMENT
Medium tempo to fast

PROGRESSION VARIABLES
Same leg to alternating legs, add weights, weight position at side to shoulder height, hands held above your head

PROGRESSION 1

Without weights, stand close to the box. Step on the platform with your entire right foot and be sure that your knee is tracking accordingly over the second long toe. I prefer that you keep your hands in front of you and not on your hips. You can also use your hands and arms to help with momentum as you alternate legs and go up and down the step.

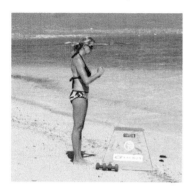 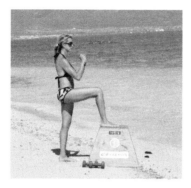 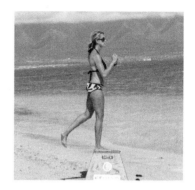

To keep the maximum strength flowing to the thigh and glute of each leg, as you step down to the ground stay close to the box. If you land too far away from the step it will result in poor form and less focused strength to the leg muscles.

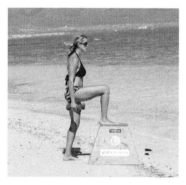 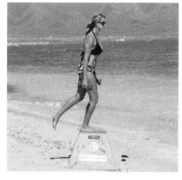 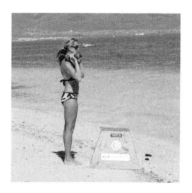

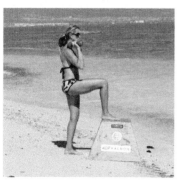 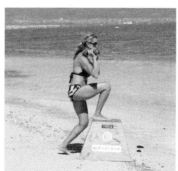 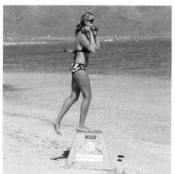

How about one set you raise your hands up above your head with your elbows bent? This will increase your cardio quite a bit. You may also do one set on the same side.

Another variable is introducing weights down at your side or resting on your shoulder. Do one set of each. Keep in mind you'll get more of a charge of strength through your body if the weights are resting on your shoulders. This is more difficult.

To add intensity, you can next choose a higher step up. You can also reverse the order from high step to low step. Changing the variables will prevent you from getting bored and will help avoid hitting training plateaus. I'll talk more about how to put this all together in programming, in Chapter 8.

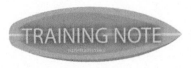
Please do not hold weights above your head as it may cause neck and/or lower back injury. I'll show you a way in Chapter 6 to combine this move with weights above your head as you learn more about cardio training for SUP.

Exercise 4:
ALTERNATING WALKING LUNGES

Walking lunges are nothing new but they build solid strength in your legs, through and through, which can translate to your SUP strength as well. I really want you to pay attention to your form, posture and knee tracking over that second long toe again. Once you nail this you can move onto the other progressions the same way.

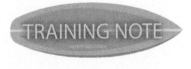
Maintain good posture throughout the exercise with shoulder blades retracted and depressed, good stability through the abdominal complex, and neutral spine angles.

SUGGESTED TRAINING EQUIPMENT
5-15 pound dumbbells

SUGGESTED REPS/SETS
20-25 reps, 1-2 sets, continuous and controlled

PROGRESSION VARIABLES
Add weights

Starting with a tall posture, feet about 3-4 inches apart and your hands clasped in front of you or with your hands on your hips, step forward with your right leg. Make sure your toes are pointed forward.

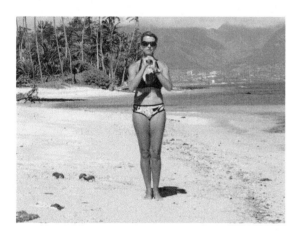 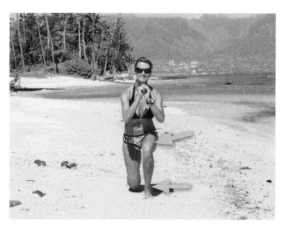

While maintaining total body alignment, step forward, descending slowly by bending at the hips, knees, and ankles. Keep most of your weight in the forward leg and AVOID letting your back knee touch the ground.

As you rise up to begin your next lunge, use your hip and thigh muscles to push yourself up and feel the momentum drive through the bottom of your heel all the way to your glute as you join the other foot. Now descend with the left leg, and repeat as you did with the first lunge again on the right and so forth.

To increase the intensity you may add dumbbells. Hold them to the side or rest them up on the shoulders as you did while doing squats.

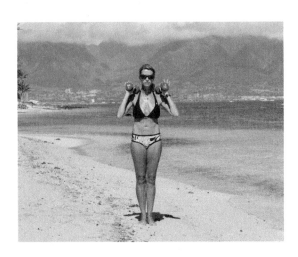
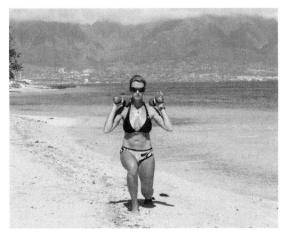

Exercise 5:
DYNAMIC SINGLE LEG SPLIT LUNGES ON CHALLENGING PLATFORM

Just when you think lunges could not get anymore exciting, I'm here to tell you that if you've ever accidentally stepped off the back of your board or even have stepped maybe too far forward off the nose and danced right off into the water, it can leave you frustrated and maybe a little embarrassed? I've actually done both. Shake it off but pay attention that you may not be as strong-legged as you think.

These exercises are for you to help you build your "dynamic" leg strength. You will use the strength you gain whenever you make simple transitions with your feet from regular stance on your board to surf stance, or when you're purposely stepping back and then back *again* on a long downwind board and don't want to get your hair wet.

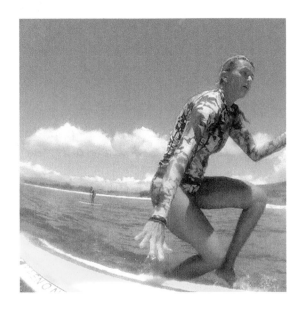

You really shouldn't have to look where your feet go on the board. It should just happen. I often have to remind my students, while on the water, to "keep looking forward."

This type of lunge is demanding and, at first, I want you to look where you plant your feet because I want your form to be perfect. The action extends and involves all joints of the leg: ankle, knee and hip. It is also good for the finer muscles.

Each platform will respond differently. For example, the BOSU offers 4 –way action and requires the foot and ankle to stabilize the entire leg throughout the movement. The half foam roller is 2-way—medial and lateral or left and right—but still offers its own unique test.

For some of the following progressions you'll definitely have to look at your feet and for others, in time, your goal should be to not have to look.

**I also highly suggest you perform these with shoes and, as with other challenging exercises, we'll start with the easiest version, progressing to the most difficult.

SUGGESTED TRAINING EQUIPMENT
5-15 pounds dumbbells, BOSU, half foam roller, Indo Board of choice, 24" Gigante Flo Cushion, full length mirror

SUGGESTED REPS/SETS
12-15, 1-2 sets

MOVEMENT
Slow and controlled with 2-5 second holds

PROGRESSION VARIABLES
Hold time, inflation percentage (%) of BOSU and Gigante Flo Cushion, add weights, board position vertically/horizontally

PROGRESSION 1

In front of the mirror place BOSU dome side up and stand about 2-3 feet away from it. Place your left foot out at a slight angle to the left. With your hands cupped together in front of you, extend your right leg into a forward lunge and place the arch of your foot directly on top of the BOSU. Be sure when you land that your knee is tracking over the second long toe.

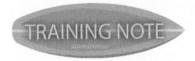

It's really important for you to keep your posture upright and don't lean or bend at the hip when you drop into your lunge.

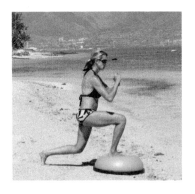 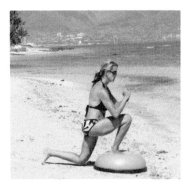 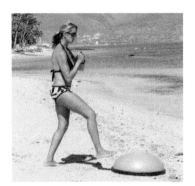

Stabilize for a few seconds and drive off the BOSU with your foot, thigh and hip to the start position. DO NOT switch sides. Repeat with good form until you've completed a full set. Then switch to the left side.

I like to add dumbbells so I can really feel the intensity and load to my butt and thigh. You can reach a little more forward with your dumbbells to find the position that makes the exercise as intense as you like.

You may also adjust your dumbbell position as you've done before and increase your hold time. With dumbbells held at your side or above the shoulder, press off back to start. This should be as smooth as your lunge. If you can't perform a repetition with a smooth return, consider reducing the amount of weight you're holding until your form is perfect. Compensation in your form is not advised.

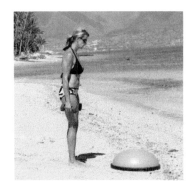 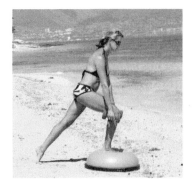 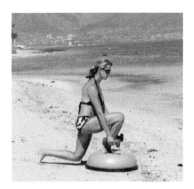

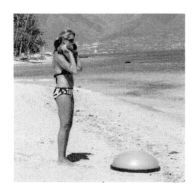 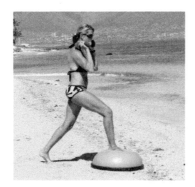 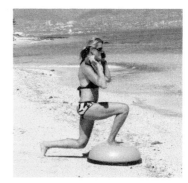

PROGRESSION 2

Performing this exercise on the Gigante Flo Cushion with your Indo Board of Choice is a blast. You can reduce the amount of inflation as a variable challenge. Even though we'll be lunging forward onto a flat board, the cushion is still considered a 4-way action platform.

This progression also requires excellent posture and proper knee tracking over the second long toe, so perform in front of the mirror. It's also tricky pressing off from your lunge back to start. Be patient and go slow. The results are worth it.

Your preparation is the same as for the former progressions. Use the widest Indo Board you have or select the easier execution. I, of course, choose the Pro Kicktail but I also have pictured here the Rocker Board. Because I have two Gigante Flo Cushions, I'll set up two and switch back and forth.

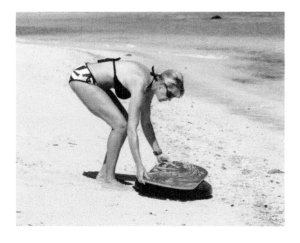 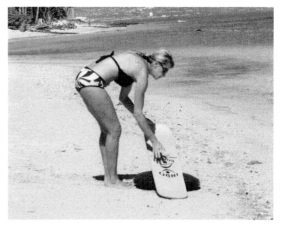

For your first few sets, position the board vertically, nose to tail with the Gigante Flo Cushion nubby side up. Once you have good execution with smooth control you can then attempt to position your board **horizontally**. It's much more difficult with the board placed horizontally.

For example, I'll start with the Rocker board for right and left leg lunges, and then switch the variable to the Pro Kicktail.

The press off from this lunge and back to the start positions is also challenging. Like the other progressions, it's best to go slow with excellent form especially when you had weights.

This concludes this chapter on ways to increase your leg strength for stand up paddling. As your legs become stronger, pay attention to the changes in your SUP performance, including your leg endurance. You might also be experiencing better paddle surfing and new, amazing pivot turns around the buoy.

You have much to work on and lots and lots of progressions to perfect. Remember to take your time and make sure each rep counts. Poor form on any of these exercises could possibly result in muscle imbalances on land that could also translate to less than stellar performance on the water.

Stay tuned next to pump it up, the heart pump that is. Chapter 6 is all about your rising heart rate performance to help you cross the finish line first.

CHAPTER 6
Cardio: The Critical Factor for All SUP Paddlers

- Why cardio is a huge factor for stronger stand up paddling.
- Is your heart ready to step up your performance?
- How does cardio affect your paddling performance?
- Learn how to test and measure your cardio fitness level.
- How to attain the SUPreme state of performance.
- Training tips/workouts to increase your heart's capacity to stronger paddling.
- Sample cardio programs.

If you've come to this chapter and are still reading this sentence, I applaud you. KEEP READING. Some call it cardio, others aerobics, vascular endurance, or physiological torture but this is probably the most important chapter of this book.

Repeat after me:
"Cardio is my friend. I love cardio. Cardio is FUN. I will be a stronger, faster paddler and will achieve a SUPreme state of paddling performance if I perform more cardio."

This section is going to help you build a stronger heart that will help you catch more waves, increase endurance for distance paddling, and virtually help you explode to a higher level of paddling performance.

The main objective is expend as little energy as possible while paddling at high levels of demand. Luckily, our bodies are very adaptable to learn how to streamline physical and mental stress over time, therefore once your heart system increases its capacity you will be able to paddle with less energy.

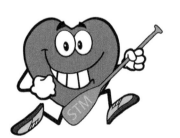

Whether you're entering your first race, or simply want to keep up with your friends so they don't leave you in the wake, it's time to put your head down, breathe and REALLY dig in. Try not to puke up a lung.

Pulse check: Do you have the heart power to help you paddle your way to the front of pack or to dodge a wall of water that is about ready to come down on your head?

Do you know what your max heart rate is? Do you have any clue what percentage of your max heart rate you should be paddling in to help preserve your energy during a distance race?

If you're a beginner to paddling you're discovering many new things, including the cardio effort required by your body to paddle. You're probably figuring out that you have to ramp up your cardio training.

Many people cringe when it comes to cardio training, but because you're serious about building max paddle stroke so you don't have a stroke, this is how your heavy breathing pays off:

Maximum Heart = Maximum Glides, Waves, Wins = Maximum Fun

You can choose to make it really complicated or not. It's that simple. As your heart capacity starts to enlarge so will the entire scope of your stand up paddling skills. The hard work you do on cardio will reward you on and off the water for many strokes and glides to come. *(At the end of the chapter there are helpful definitions of terms that are used throughout this chapter.)*

How well you become connected to your heart stress levels and percentages of your heart rate will translate into your paddling efficiency. This may be a real wake up call as you start examining your true SUP fitness. You may have incredible upper body or leg strength, but how 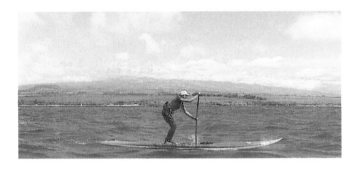 well do you perform at the start of a sprint race and how well can you manage your cardio stress throughout?

EXAMPLES OF HOW CARDIO PLAYS A KEY ROLE IN YOUR SUP PERFORMANCE

A little while back I wrote an article called *Downwind Stand Up Paddling Requires a Big Heart.* In the article I mentioned that downwind paddling requires a big lung capacity because it's like interval sprint paddling. Some moments you're hunkered down paddling against big side swells and side chop just to get out to the start of the downwinder. Then the other times you have to paddle fast and hard with explosive strokes to catch the bumps and glides. You repeat that process for 10 miles.

I often have the pleasure of training many amazing endurance athletes. On the mainland they are naturals to flat-water paddling and do very well very quickly because their lung capacity is already trained. You can spot these folks pretty fast. But, the moment I get them in big open ocean swell, their adrenaline is surging and presenting in ways they've never experienced, causing very erratic heart rate transitions that are hard to manage.

One year I had a very fit guy just about bonk on me one day while paddling his first Maliko downwind adventure. He prepared and paddled on the mainland and performed the exercises I suggested via SKYPE. When he arrived, we also had time to review his training on land. We also did a couple mini downwinders first and I felt he was well prepared and ready to rock.

About five minutes into the paddle, the moment he got out to the first set of rocks where the reef starts to feather, he realized this was very different than the lakes back home; his whole body shook. He had reached his anaerobic threshold or AT which is NOT how you want to start your first Maliko downwind run! (Refer to definitions at the end of this article.)

The energy he spent in this state caused his heart rate to sore near his max and it stayed there for about 4 miles. This is not a good thing and not at all what he is used to. It took us about 30 minutes of sitting and talking story and chilling, while I watched him like a hawk and kept him calm. He was a little embarrassed and said, "This never happens."

My goal for him at that moment was to get his heart rate down so we could continue on safely. He was blown away at how his heart rate increased so fast—particularly because he was a fine tuned machine, so he could normally perform at lower heart rate percentage, which is the ideal physiological state.

Another example is for the wave paddlers out there. Having great big lungs to hold your breath for the unforeseen hold-downs takes time to build. Training for this includes lots of practice and keeping calm. I know that the top guys SUP paddling into JAWS have their heart rates wired to the single beat. A lot of them also take up free-diving as a way to train to hold their breath for long periods of time.

About two years ago I was out at one of our local breaks and it was super big. I was pretty on it that day and felt strong and had a good rhythm going of catching some bombs, resting on the shoulder, and then going in for some more.

There are some days when a sneaker set comes along and takes out everyone in the lineup which is actually great, because if you time it right, you're not in that lineup, you're in the one just outside and then your path is cleared! The next wave is yours.

Then you have to choose a line that won't fold over or close out. You just go and hope for the best. This time I was caught off guard and it closed out from behind. It was like a heavy, big tall building falling down on me and I didn't see it coming, but I sure heard it.

Normally the sound is enough to peel you out of your skin, but it happened so fast I just thought, "Whoa, this is cool, I'm surfing." Then, "BOOM." I thought someone took a swing at the back of my head with what felt like a 2 by 4 piece of wood. Then the "fun" began.

Somehow I managed not to get tangled in my leash and I tried with all my might to not let my paddle punch me in the nose. Sometimes it can also be best to toss your paddle. I was getting worked and worked and worked. I looked up and *thought* the light was near—my path out to take a breath before the next beating.

Here is what the event looked like from my Go Pro on the North Shore of Maui:

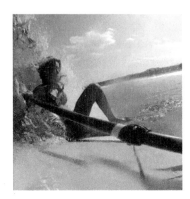 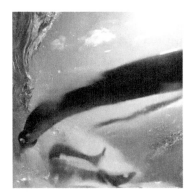 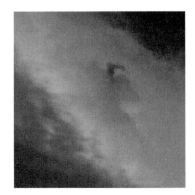

The board and I took a big spin in the rinse cycle. You can see just my foot as the wave twisted and spun.

Unfortunately, it was an ambient light reflection of white foam about 4 feet deep. I stupidly took a breath and sucked in the ocean. Then I started to panic a little. I was losing my lung capacity, and, I thought, my life.

I got tossed around again and finally came up. I was pushed back in to shore far enough in that I wasn't in anyone's way. It was just me; hacking up a lung and maybe a turtle. I never in my life coughed that hard and then I couldn't stop for 3 hours after I made it in. I went to the hospital to be sure I didn't have secondary drowning. My lungs were clear but they burned for days.

It was extra motivation for me to increase my lung capacity, and it was also a time to reflect how important it is to be humble and maybe not push my luck. I've realized every time I place myself in those situations that I had better feel strong enough not only in my body but also in my heart, literally.

These are maybe extreme examples of situations you may find yourself in as you begin to increase your strength and skills in your stand up paddling performance, but hopefully you see my point.

Of all the paddlers I've met around the world, what impresses me most are those that seem to be born with amazing lungs. Sure, they also train hard and make it look easy. I'm talking about the SUP athletes who are strong off the start of a sprint or distance race, and are the same SUP athletes that are able to keep it together and not blow up. I admire that because that is not my strongest SUP performance skill. I personally must have been born with small lungs but I keep at it, building my capacity.

There is something to be said for the hereditary attributes of this amazing, unique athletic ability, as it is certainly true. Some people are born with great cardio endurance and others have to work very hard at developing it. Also, you may notice after a day or week or month of slacking off on your training, it can feel like you're starting all over again at ground zero when you pick back up again.

When you can fine-tune your rhythm, from the beat of your heart to the cadence of your paddle speed, and manage your cadence all throughout any type of race course, you will have reached the ultimate in SUP cardio performance.

I often say,

"As you begin to get more comfortable being uncomfortable during your cardio training, that's when the real adaptation and stimulation starts in your cardiovascular system."

HOW MUCH DO YOU KNOW ABOUT YOUR HEART STRENGTH?

The more you know about the heart system and how to measure your own cardio stress, the easier it will be to learn how to train more effectively on and off the water. I'd like you to start thinking about cardio as part your regular training—in addition to the balance and strength training. You have to do all three if you want to achieve a "SUPreme" state of performance.

When I ask clients how they perceive "really" working hard versus *my* version of really working hard, it's not uncommon for people to underestimate their perceived level of heart work by 50% or more.

For example, their perceived level of exertion or paddling in technical speak of a scale of 1-10 may seem like a 9 or even 10, but when I test them for the same task we're talking a 3 or 4. See the illustration below.

Perceived Level of Exertion

I've developed this illustration specifically for stand up paddling. It is a simple way to gauge your cardio work levels by simply rating yourself without a heart rate monitor. But, as I mentioned, you may think you're really working hard but if I was next to you we may discover your 9 is my 4. Please keep in mind that your age, level of fitness, chronic diseases, physical conditions, and medications can affect how you feel.

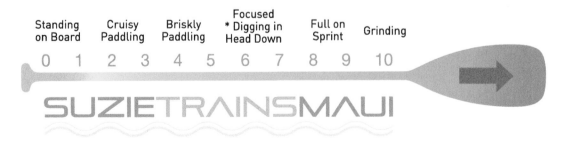

PERCEIVED LEVEL OF EXERTION WHILE STAND UP PADDLING

Standing on Board	Cruisy Paddling	Briskly Paddling	Focused * Digging in Head Down	Full on Sprint	Grinding
0 1	2 3	4 5	6 7	8 9	10

SUZIETRAINSMAUI

Using this illustration is a nice way to keep yourself in check as you begin your cardio training for stand up paddling. The key principal is to make note of how your body responds as you progress through this scale.

Start thinking about where your cardio strength is now, in relation to the chart. If you're a beginner paddler could you manage to be in the "4 or 5" zone level of effort for 5 minutes without rest? Or, if you're an advanced paddler can you maintain an "8" for effort for say 5, 8 and then 10 minutes? It's fun to see how long you can go.

What you could try as you get more comfortable with cardio, or if you're already pro, is to set yourself up for a mini cardio paddling interval blast. For example you'd paddle into zone 9-10 for 30 seconds, rest for 30, then again for 45 seconds with a 30 second rest, then a full one minute paddling frenzy with a few minutes rest. Repeat several times. I'd love to hear how you do!

I recommend now to go out and do a test paddle to see where you think you are on this chart. Be very honest with yourself. With this new level of understanding as to where your heart strength might be, our next step is to start measuring and testing it. Continue reading.

What is your heart rate and how to find and calculate it:

There are a couple of standard ways to find your pulse and heart rate. Here are two quick methods:

1. Take your right index and middle finger and place on the underside of your left wrist below the thumb. Do not use your right thumb to take your pulse. Apply gentle pressure on your left wrist and you should be able to feel your pulse. You may need to move your fingers around a bit to find it. This is known as your radial pulse.

2. Another way to discover your pulse is to take the same two fingers of the right hand and press just underneath the rear line of your jaw of your neck. Apply gentle pressure to search for your pulse. This is also known as the carotid pulse method because this is where your carotid artery is located.

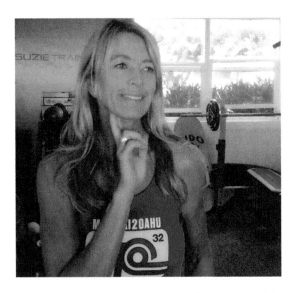 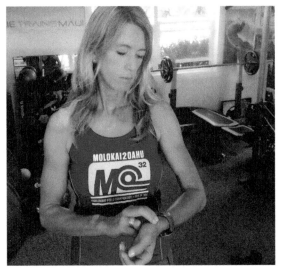

Now simply use a watch with a second hand, or look at a clock with a second hand. Count the beats you feel for 10 seconds. Multiply this number by six to get your heart rate (pulse) per minute.

Count your pulse: _____ beats in 10 seconds x 6 = _____ beats/minute

What is a normal resting pulse?

Normal Heart Rates at Rest:

- Children (ages 6 - 15) 70 – 100 beats per minute
- Adults (age 18 and over) 60 – 100 beats per minute
- Hear rate at rest for top elite athletes: 40-60 beats per minute (Males will have slightly lower resting heart rate than females.)

Generally, a lower heart rate at rest implies more efficient heart function and better cardiovascular fitness. For example, a well-trained paddler might have a normal resting heart rate closer to 40 beats per minute. For men, the average resting heart rate is between 70 and 72 beats per minute, and for women it is usually between 78 and 82 bpm.

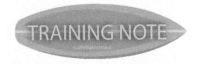 *It takes fewer heartbeats to power a well-conditioned SUP athlete during intense training as well as during rest.*

You can start by recording your heart rate before your paddle, during and after and learn how your heart responds to different levels of paddling exertion.

Soon you will outgrow the chart and method above and will want to know your average heart rate and your max heart rate. At that point it's time to get a heart rate monitor.

I promise you, if you begin to start monitoring your heart rate during a warm up, during your max effort and most importantly, during your cool-down, your SUP cardio performance will rise.

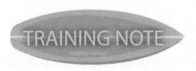

How fast you can recover and bring your heart rate down from an event is almost more important how you perform during the event. The disciplined practice of recovery could land you a nice spot on the podium too.

Discovering More About Your Heart Rate

Next we'll talk about **Max HR**, or Maximum Heart Rate, and **Target HR**. This is where your body is pushed to the max and the state of your cardio workout becomes less aerobic to, even, anaerobic at times. Knowing the basics about this is important so stay with me. (Refer to terms at end of this chapter.)

Your maximum heart rate is the highest heart rate achieved during maximal exercise and when you are in a full on grind. Although there are many formulas to determine your max heart rate, I recommend using the formula below. (Keep in mind there can be some region of error of 10-20 beats per minute and may be inaccurate for those already high-level paddlers.) Most heart rate monitors will use this calculation as well.

220 - your age **= predicted maximum heart rate**

If you are more active and have been exercising for a while, use the 205 – your age**.**

Example: a 40-year-old's predicted maximum heart rate is 180 beats/minute.

Knowing your maximum heart rate while you're paddling will help you find a target range or ideal range for your pulse during your paddling and/or training session. Exercising above 90 percent of your MHR moves your body from aerobic exercise (with oxygen) into anaerobic exercise (without oxygen).

Going a little deeper, it's important to know that the average person can't sustain paddling or training at this level (anaerobic) for more than a minute or two. During anaerobic activity the body mainly depends on glycogen storage from the muscles for fuel instead of using the more efficient methods of aerobic training. You'll quickly end up with a buildup of waste products in the bloodstream that will overtake the healthy blood you need.

You may have heard of the term lactic acid, which is a common byproduct of muscle metabolism. Too much of this glucose breaking down and building up in your body and you can suffer dearly with muscle burning and a drought of energy, which could cause you to pull out of a race. It's also referred to as bonking.

This is why fatigue can quickly set in after you sprint off the start and paddle too hot and too hard. Your body can't operate at this level and is searching for it's normal, aerobic state.

To make sure we keep you paddling in an *aerobic* state it's good to know your **target heart rate**. I'm not going to get heavy on "zone" training I just want you to someday know by feel how to plan your paddling and cardio to work your heart appropriately. These are just some of the tools to help you build this heart awareness as your stand up paddling performance improves.

Here are the numbers on where you can start with your target heart rate. The table below shows estimated target heart rates for different ages. In the age category closest to yours, read across to find your target heart rate. If we know your maximum heart rate is approximately 220 minus your age. The figures are averages, so use them as general guidelines. (Note: this chart does not apply to those using the formula of 205 –age)

Age	Target HR Zone 50-85%	Average Maximum Heart Rate, 100%
20 years	100-170 beats per minute	200 beats per minute
30 years	95-162 beats per minute	190 beats per minute
35 years	93-157 beats per minute	185 beats per minute
40 years	90-153 beats per minute	180 beats per minute
45 years	88-149 beats per minute	175 beats per minute
50 years	85-145 beats per minute	170 beats per minute
55 years	83-140 beats per minute	165 beats per minute
60 years	80-136 beats per minute	160 beats per minute
65 years	78-132 beats per minute	155 beats per minute
70 years	75-128 beats per minute	150 beats per minute

So how can you use this target heart rate guide for your SUP cardio training?

If you're paddling in a target heart rate that is too high, you're going to spend too much energy too soon. Best to slow your cadence down a bit and find a sustaining a percentage that's just on the borderline of being uncomfortable, but one you can control.

However if you're paddling too slow and your work and speed is too slow, and the intensity feels "light" or "moderate/brisk," push yourself to paddle and dig in a little harder.

Keep your breath steady with controlled breathing. Develop a rhythm between your stroke and your breaths that feels efficient and manageable. When things get tough on the water, I really tune into this to help me regain my focus and hold my course. As my speed and cadence increases I'll push short, fast breaths out.

After an explosive 30-45 seconds all out grind to catch up to someone and pass them, I'll exhale 1-3 big breaths to help re-regulate my heart rate back to a state of aerobic energy. Then I can look for the next person to pass!

When I'm training for races I'm very aware of my heart rate. I look to see where my average is now and then just to check in to see if what I'm feeling is on track. I can set my Garmin to 4 fields and see at all times how hard I'm working or not. If I'm slacking, I pump it up. It's helpful for me to able to adjust this as I'm paddling. I then go home and download my data to see what my actuals were at certain parts of my paddle session. I can usually recall feeling specific upticks and drops in my heart rate that correspond to the data output.

For example, if I'm approaching a very sticky or slow section and the wind dies and the current is moving in a non-favorable direction, you can bet I'll be working that much harder. I can pinpoint on my GPS map exactly where I was at that time. It's very cool.

Here's an example of what my heart rate looked like during a very difficult "no wind," hot, humid, downwind race in May of 2014.

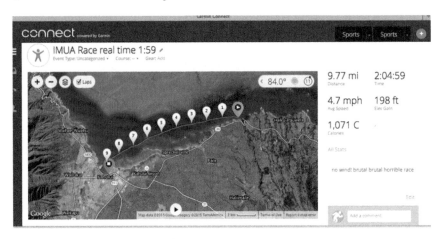

This is our usual course where my average speed on a 14 foot board is usually 12-15 miles per hour and I'm averaging 9 minute miles. During this race my time splits were more like 12 minute miles. I counted three glides the entire race with a max speed of 9mph. (Not fun!)

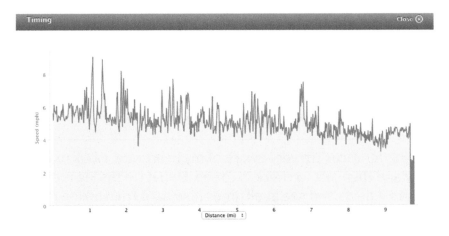

How to Increase Your Stand Up Paddling Performance

My max heart rate when I'm "working hard" in primo conditions is 162 and my average is roughly 130 beats per minute. So I'm working but not dying.

HOWEVER during this race check out my heart rate! My average was my max at 172 and then my "max" was 183 on a couple occasions. Not good. I burned over a thousand calories and barely had enough water. I thought my head was going to pop off my body. Some paddlers pulled out of the race. Where my heart was peaking is when I would go for any bump. I'd sprint then glide. The final peak is at the mouth of the harbor and then the slow grind to the finish inside.

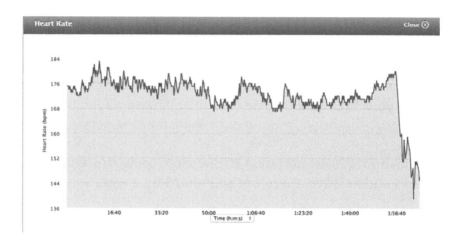

During the first few weeks of working out and paddling, I suggest you aim for the lowest part of your target zone (50 percent). Then, gradually build up to the higher part (85 percent). You might even get so good at this you can count the number of strokes per minute that will match your percentage of your max heart rate. If you can get that tuned in please let me know so I can brag about you!

As you begin to build even better cardio endurance for your stand up paddling, say after 5-6 months, you may be able to paddle comfortably at up to 85 percent of your maximum heart rate. But you don't have to paddle or exercise that hard all the time to stay in great cardio shape. Remember, your body only has so much total capacity to give you and you must have some energy left in reserve. Just like your car, driving around on empty or near empty, dirties your fuel filter. Don't dirty your body; save some for later when you may need a clean, hard push.

According to Dr. Hirofumi Tanaka, PhD, associate professor of kinesiology and health education at the University of Texas and director of the university's

Cardiovascular Aging Research Laboratory, "Whether you're a couch potato or a highly trained athlete, that rate declines about seven beats per minute for each decade."

Since we're talking numbers, it's important for me to tell you not to get too fixated on them. Keep in mind that every "body" is unique and like your age, your current state of health or different types of medication you may be taking can affect your heart rate and your training capacity. Always be sure to notify your physician if you don't feel right or have questions about your physical health and wellness.

TRANSITIONING FROM SUPER TO SUPERIOR SUP PADDLING PERFORMANCE

Put on your snorkel right here and go a bit deeper with me if you really want to learn about how to maximize your heart performance for SUP like the elite paddlers. Getting your **VO2 Max** measured is the ultimate way to help you learn how you tolerate high intensity paddling or training for long periods of time.

Your goal is to have your heart pumping efficiently to bring fresh blood throughout your body to cells and muscles, therefore spending less energy with every stroke.

Knowing your VO2Max values is good information to have so you can determine *how efficiently* your body consumes and absorbs oxygen while grinding in the red paddle zone, as well while you're paddling at other levels of exertion. (Refer to chart above.) This is called VO2 Max training.

VO2Max refers to the maximum amount of oxygen that an individual can utilize during intense or maximal exercise. It is measured as "milliliters" of oxygen used during one minute per kilogram of body weight.

The very best way of getting this measured is being in a controlled environment with a specialist directly testing you as you inhale and exhale at different levels of intensity and speed. You will be max tested on a treadmill or spin bike for about 10-15 minutes to your complete max. Just a warning—this process can be very painful. Before you go there, make sure your technician is well qualified and prepares you in advance on what to expect and how hard you are expected to push.

You'll be asked to wear a mask that captures all exhalations, and then measures the amount of oxygen and carbon dioxide that is being exhaled to calculate how much oxygen you are actually using. This is where your body is forced to go into that state from using oxygen or aerobic energy metabolic system and cross over to the anaerobic metabolic system using glycogen stores. The cost of this test can range from $75-$500, depending on where you go.

Once you've obtained this information and norm values you can then determine how to best approach and adjust your training to achieve your maximum SUP performance.

Keep in mind, like all SUP races, divisions and levels of paddlers, there are variables that affect your maximum cardio potential. In review, those things are:

Genetic factors, Age, Gender, and Altitude

For example it's been observed that elite females have a higher V02Max level than men. Although, due to a male's body composition and other physiological differences, a non-elite athlete women's V02Max is generally lower.

Age has a real effect on one's SUP performance and cardio potential. In general, VO2 max is the highest at age **20** and decreases nearly 30 percent by age 65. Yikes!

People will often "altitude" train to help boost their V02 values because there is less oxygen at higher altitudes. That means an athlete will generally have a 5 percent decrease in VO2 max results with a 5,000 feet gain in altitude.

Simple Tests to Measure Your VO2 Max

There are many ways and formulas that are used to measure your VO2 Max without the fancy machines. You can also search online for quick collective computer models into which you can simply enter data. I've selected to the most common two.

Use the simple V02 Max **Rockport Test** if you're not as fit. If you're pretty fit you can select **The Cooper's Test**.

Rockport VO2 Max Test: Consists of walking on a treadmill or outside as fast as you can for one mile.

What you need for the Rockport VO2 Max Test: Stopwatch or watch, treadmill or outdoor track that equals one (1) mile. You can also use a fancy heart rate monitor that can do all of these tasks except do the test for you. I the Garmin Forerunner 310 XT.

- Record your weight.
- Walk on a treadmill with no grade increase as fast as possible. Do not run or jog. Complete your walk as fast as possible outside and record your time.

Immediately record your heart beats for 1 minute. Or to simplify like you learned earlier in this chapter:

Count the beats you feel for 10 seconds. Multiply this number by six to get your heart rate (pulse) per minute.

Count your pulse: _____ beats in 10 seconds x 6 = _____ beats/minutes

The formula for estimating that peak aerobic capacity:

Estimated VO2 max (ml/kg/min) = 132.853 - (0.0769 x body weight in [pounds]) - (0.3877 x age [years]) + (6.3150 x gender [female = 0; male = 1]) - (3.2649 x 1-mile walk time [in minutes and hundredths]) - (0.1565 x 1-minute heart rate at end of mile [beats per minute]).

Results are expressed as: ml/kg/min

Note: On the basis of the validity (R=.88) and standard error of estimate (5.0 ml/kg/min), you can be about 68% sure that your true VO2 max is ± 5.0 ml/kg/min of your calculated value. For example, if your predicted VO2 max is 40 ml/kg/min, there is a 68% likelihood that your actual value is between 35 and 45.

V02 Max Aerobic Capacity Norms			
Values expressed in ml/kg/min			
Age	Fitness Levels	Males	Females
20-29	Low Fitness	<37.1	<30.6
	Moderately Fit	37.1 -44.2	30.6 – 36.6
	High Fitness	44.3+	36.7+
30-39	Low Fitness	<35.3	<28.7
	Moderately Fit	35.3 -42.4	28.7 – 34.6
	High Fitness	42.5+	34.7+
40-49	Low Fitness	<33.0	<26.0
	Moderately Fit	33.0 – 39.9	26.5 -32.3
	High Fitness	40.0+	32.4+
50-59	Low Fitness	<31.4	<25.1
	Moderately Fit	31.4 – 39.3	25.1 – 31.3
	High Fitness	39.4+	31.4+
Ages 60+	Low Fitness	<28.3	<21.9
	Moderately Fit	28.3 – 36.1	21.9 – 28.2
	High Fitness	36.2+	28.3+

The second test you can perform as you become more fit is called the **Cooper Test**. It consists of running as fast as you can as far as you can in 12 minutes.

The Cooper test was developed in the 1960's by Dr. Kenneth Cooper, which is still the standard cardio test in the military. To this day, it is a commonly used test to measure VO2 Max. The biggest advantage being that it is the most simple to perform without much assistance or expense.

Cooper's VO2 max estimation formula depends solely on the *distance* covered during 12 minutes of sustained running. Here, distance is measured in meters and VO2 max is measured in mL/kg/min. (You may need to convert your miles to meters.) The formula is:

VO_2 Max = (D - 504.9)/44.73, where D is the distance run (in meters) during 12 minutes.

What you need: An outdoor track or area marked at .25 mile intervals, or you may also wear a heart rate monitor/GPS watch that tracks your distance in meters so you don't have to convert afterward.

For Example: Sarah SUP warms up for 2-3 minutes and then times herself for 12 minutes while running. At the end of 12 minutes she has run 1.75 miles (7 laps around a track). Since 1.75 miles = 2816 meters, she can estimate her VO_2 by computing the below:

Sarah SUP's VO_2 Max = (2816 - 504.9)/44.73 = **51.67 mL/kg/min**.

Here are the results: (as mentioned you will have to find an online converter to Convert miles to meters)

Cooper Test (Experienced Athletes)					
	Excellent	**Good**	**Average**	**Bad**	**Poor**
Male	3700+ m	3400 - 3700 m	3100 - 3399 m	2800 - 3099 m	2800- m
Female	3000+ m	2700 - 3000 m	2400 - 2699 m	2100 - 2399 m	2100- m

As you begin to discover your own cardio capacity you will need to maintain it on a regular basis, learn how to manage and recognize if you are pushing too hard, and set realistic goals to increase it.

Everyone is unique in how his or her body adapts to cardio stress. It takes time to make changes. Be sure to hydrate well and fuel your body when attempting to elevate your cardio fitness. Be sure to check out my tips on nutrition and fueling in Chapter 10.

TRAINING TIPS TO BOOST YOUR CARDIO PERFORMANCE FOR SUP

Fun & Simple: First, it must be **fun**. Select a type of exercise that you will "enjoy" and that you are psyched to get out and do. Be realistic of your real fitness currently as you want to set yourself up for success.

Next keep it simple. Just like the acronym KISS I'm sure you've heard at least once or twice in your life, keep it simple well, normally I'd say stupid, but here I'll interject super. SUPER!

By keeping it **simple**, I mean start out with a simple approach like adding interval sprints to your morning jog. Or check out a spin class or two, hop on a mountain bike or road bike, or, even better, get out on the water and practice interval sprints on your board.

What you're doing here is introducing new **variables** to current routines. Slowly they will become a new standard and slowly your heart capacity will also expand. It's also important to mix it up. So pick a few different exercises.

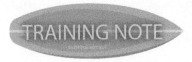 *Did you know swimming one mile is equivalent to running 4 miles? Go swim.*

Another tip that really motivates my clients and me is the act of putting on a heart rate monitor, hitting the start button and seeing what we've got. Being purposeful in your action of improving your cardio is a great way to learn more about your body. You'll discover what it feels like when training at 70% of your max versus 90% of your max heart rate. Now this is real, not your own perceived level of exertion. Remember the colored paddle above that illustrates paddle cardio effort.

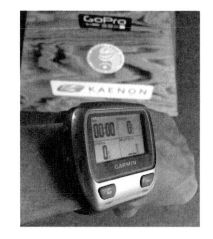

It also serves as a great way to literally track your progress of how fast and how hard you have to work to get to your max and how fast you recover. The software that comes with some of the heart rate monitors allows you to see elevation change, where you actually were on the water and more cool things. Look back over a week, 2 weeks and then two months. It's exciting to not only *feel* your progress, but also to see your progress.

Which brings me to a really important topic to cover, and that is to talk about getting your heart rate down to its normal resting state after you've pushed really hard. I could write an entire chapter on this but to help you adopt this concept, we'll keep it simple.

Recovery heart rate will vary based on current level of fitness, gender, age, and other genetic characteristics. During your first minute of recovery after a planned and timed cardio session your heart rate will start to drop pretty dramatically. If you are not as fit, it could take more time to drop.

More specifically, a really fit athlete's heart rate will return to a normal state in just few minutes while, for someone who is less fit, it could take two to three times longer. (Note, if it takes a dramatically long time to recover you may want to see your physician)

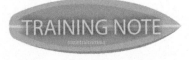

The second minute after your workout is where we can actually record your improvement and progress. Simply record your heart rate during your workout. Then after you stop, wait one minute, record, then record again at the 2-minute mark. Subtract the two-minute recovery rate from the working heart rate to determine a baseline for improvement.

So for example, if your training heart rate during exercise is 190 and your resting heart rate is 80, it could take you several minutes for your heart rate to return to normal. While your heart rate might drop about 20 beats during the first minute, it will drop at a slower rate (decreasing 15 beats per minute or so) during the second and third minutes.

Get to know your resting heart rate well and watch for any small or significant changes.

THE SUPREME STATE OF PERFORMANCE

Another component within the topic of recovery heart rate is to find a way for you to innately know how to work at a high heart rate to achieve pretty decent speed/paddling cadence during a distance race and/or during a sprint race. It's also important to learn how to control your heart rate so that it isn't high all of the time, but yet you're still able to move quickly. Remember you can't maintain 90-95% of your max heart for very long or you could bonk. But, you can paddle up to that max a few times or more during an event, depending on how fine-tuned you are.

I guess you could call it "The Zone," but that is so cliché or so I like to call it the **SUPreme state of performance**. Many sports psychologists try to explain this sort of euphoric state when an athlete's brain just clicks in as if they've checked out to a place even they cannot describe. It's an awesome reward as a trainer to see this go down.

For example, the top SUP athletes know exactly where their heart rate needs to be in this **SUPreme state of performance** in order for them to save enough heart energy so they can pass the next paddler in their line of sight and to still finish strong. They may repeat this pattern 3 or more times in one race, if they're well trained, use their head, and know their heart capacity—it can be done.

You may already have experienced lots of heart rate changes at the start of race. The jitters and butterflies already have your heart rate soring. The added surge of adrenaline combines with jockeying for position with fifty or a hundred or more people crammed next to you; the horn goes off and you go absolutely balls out. (Sorry Ladies)

Remember how that feels? Your throat is dry and you are laser focused on being in the top lead straight away. Someone may already be drafting and sucking you dry, but how is your heart rate? Is your Garmin going to explode off your wrist or are you calm, in control of your breath, and saving some for later?

After you've raced in enough races, from flat water to downwind, with all types of conditions and in many different types of weather, including heat, cold, humidity, snow, or brutal sand storms in Dubai (where you have to wear a face mask); you'll get to know your own, best personal **SUPreme state of performance** pretty quickly.

The takeaway here is to know that there is no magic heart rate number or percentage that will always be the same. You are changing everyday, every month, and every year.

I suggest you look for consistent patterns and learn how you can tweak certain things—possibly your stroke, your breathing techniques, and the way you fuel yourself to help your lungs go big.

If poor paddling technique is causing you to spend more energy than you think you should, have someone help you fine-tune your stroke. If you feel your energy is not quite right, see your physician. You may be lacking an important nutrient or have another condition that can be addressed. Of course, resting is also very important.

Rest is Key

Sometimes you need good old-fashioned rest to help recharge your mind and body. I've suggested to Kody Kerbox to go kick a soccer ball around a big open field and spend some time on land riding a mountain bike. Get your head and body off the water and hit the reset button. You'd be surprised how much this helps keep your mind clear and allows the cells and muscles of your body take a necessary pause.

Having trained a few IROMAN athletes I've seen a consistent pattern plateauing simply because they are worn down. Their cardio is often stagnating, as is their body. Training consumes them and it's their life. Sometimes simply changing your environment and doing something completely opposite of your normal routine can really help rebuild your cardio capacity once again. Give it a try.

Next up, what exactly can you do to get that heart rate ticking up? I have all sorts of suggestions for you.

WAYS TO GET YOUR TICKER TICKING

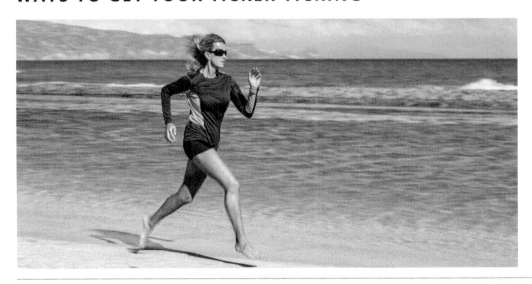

How to Increase Your Stand Up Paddling Performance

We've got a good understanding on the importance of knowing your **SUPreme state of performance**. You can keep it simple in ways I've already suggested but let's now get creative and have a little fun! Remember that word "fun."

I've listed some of the ways in which I help clients step up their heart game so they can step up their SUP game pretty quickly and in a fun and safe way.

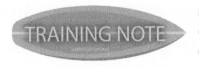 *I would like to always suggest that you can modify any exercises or workouts in this book—especially in this cardio section—to avoid injury. Go easy and go smart. Always consult with your physician.*

A few of these cardio workouts and exercises may be familiar to you. There is no special order or one that is really better than the other as they all have the same goal in mind—and that is to get your heart rate up. Try one or two or try them all.

TOTAL BODY EXERCISES

Total body exercises are designed to use your entire body and to get your heart rate up. They are usually performed at a higher rate of speed. They are fun and allow you to change many variables along the way, often training at least two or more muscle groups at the same time and including multiple joint movements.

Some place extra stress on your heart by the mere fact you are transitioning from the prone or face down position to a full upright position. Some use extra weight while others use just your own body weight.

You can change the speed or tempo in which you perform the exercise or the platform on which you train. I would caution on using light weights only. You can time yourself for 1-2 minutes (very hard) or complete 20-50 reps in 1-3 sets. Or for those of you who have a couple board plugs loose, you can go to total fatigue. LOL.

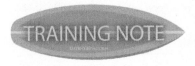 *Another cool thing to do is to raise your hands above your head on just about any exercise and watch your heart rate soar. Good luck.*

FIVE TOTAL BODY EXERCISES

Exercise 1:
SQUAT TO SHOULDER PRESS

Perform a simple squat then immediately perform a 2-arm or alternating arm shoulder press.

SUGGESTED WEIGHT
Body weight, 2-8 pounds.

SUGGESTED EQUIPMENT
Light weights—3-8 pounds, Indo Board of choice, or BOSU

SUGGESTED REPS/SETS/TIME
20-25 reps, 2-3 sets, or timed 1-2 minute sets

PROGRESSION VARIABLES
Add light weights, stand on the Indo Board of choice and Gigante Flo Cushion, time for 1-2 minutes or go for 25 reps x 2 sets, slow or fast

---

PROGRESSION 1

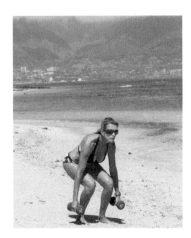 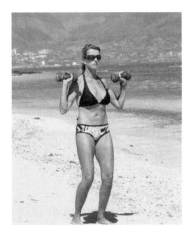 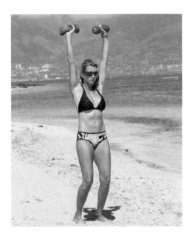

PROGRESSION 2

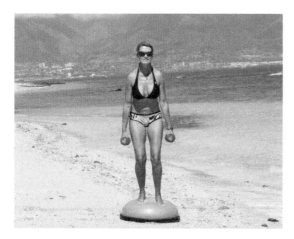 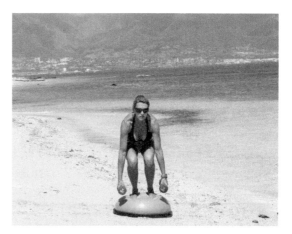

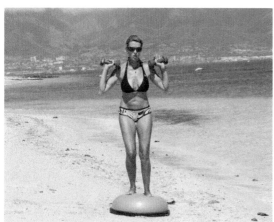 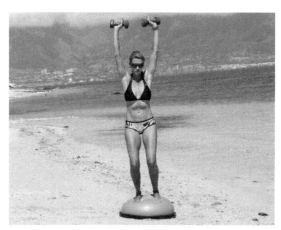

Exercise 2:
KETTLE BELL SWINGS

These are great! You must have good form so as not to hurt your lower back. Before you go all in, make sure you're doing them right.

Hold the kettle bell in front of you with two hands using a semi-light grip. With legs wide and toes pointed out at 10 & 2, bend your knees and begin to swing kettle bell through your legs. Draw in your stomach to the front of your spine.

As you come up, be sure, for sure, to **squeeze your butt cheeks** as you swing up the kettle bell to just at chin level. Don't allow the kettle bell to rise too high past your chin. As you begin the next one, keep your eyes forward at all times. Soon the natural inertia will start to flow. DON'T LET GO OF THE KETTLE BELL EVER until you are done with your set.

SUGGESTED EQUIPMENT
(1) 10-15 pound kettle bell

SUGGESTED REPS/SETS/TIME
20-25 reps, 2-3 sets, or timed 1-2 minutes

PROGRESSION VARIABLES
Shuffle across floor with kettle bell or perform what I call the "cowgirl/boy." Shuffling takes some practice and all you have to do is do a side step sort of lunge, swing and repeat. Change direction.

REGULAR

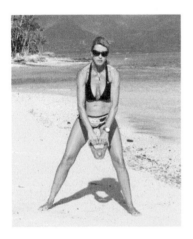 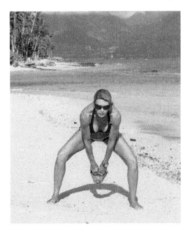 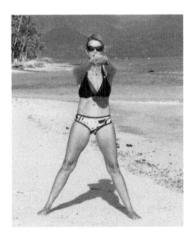

SHUFFLE

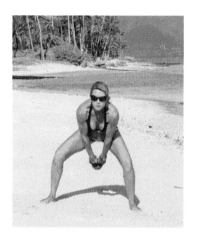 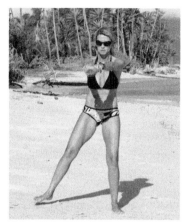 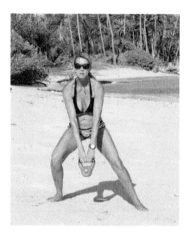

Exercise 3:
MOUNTAIN CLIMBERS

Since you'll be in the prone position or face down the entire exercise, your heart will really tick upward. Keep breathing at a steady pace. You can perform this exercise at many different tempos and with different types of equipment. Just keep moving. You can mix the variables below in different sets as well.

Place hands on the floor with your legs extended behind you. As you alternate legs, bring your knee to your chest, return, and keep going. It's a kind of running motion, but horizontal. Keep your abs drawn in.

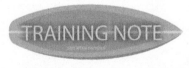

TRAINING NOTE

You'll want to avoid possible dizziness. Once you are in the prone position for an extended period of time, you'll be working quite hard. When you have completed your set, please rise up very slowly as you return to a standing state. I do this when I train by counting slowly 1, 2, 3.

SUGGESTED EQUIPMENT
Floor, the fixed perfect push up bars, BOSU

SUGGESTED REPS/SETS/TIME
20-25 reps, 2-3 sets, or timed 1-2 minutes

PROGRESSION VARIABLES
I like to use the perfect push up bars so I can really go fast. They keep my wrists from hurting. For an added challenge you can turn a BOSU upside down. Be sure your chest is aligned over the white plug and your hands are placed on the outside handles. You can also place your hands atop of an Indo Board while it's placed on top of the Gigante Flo Cushion.

You can also perform this exercise fast like a scissors split with added hop, if you will, alternate legs and be sure to maintain contact with the ground. I love doing these!

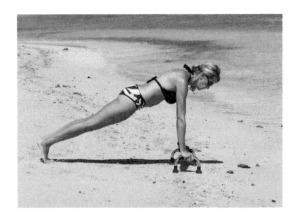 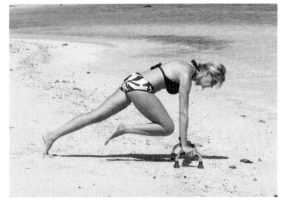

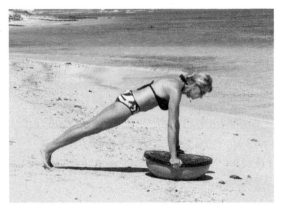 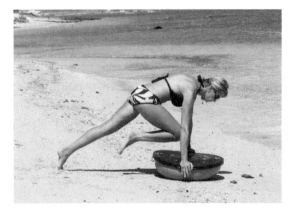

Exercise 4:
SPLIT LUNGE TWO ARM BICEP CURL

This should be performed with light weights.

Begin with both feet shoulder width apart and hold two dumbbells in your hands at chest level you're your palms facing your body. Lunge forward, landing on the heel. Make sure your knee is aligned over your second long toe. Perform a bicep curl.

SUGGESTED EQUIPMENT
Light weights: 5-10 pound dumbbells

SUGGESTED REPS/SETS/TIME
20-25 reps, 2-3 sets, or timed 1-2 minutes

PROGRESSION VARIABLES
Perform regular or hammer curls

While in the lunge position drive off the front foot (heel first) and back into a standing position, bringing your hands and dumbbells back up to the chest with palms facing toward you. Switch to the other leg and continue.

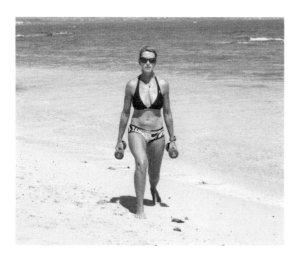
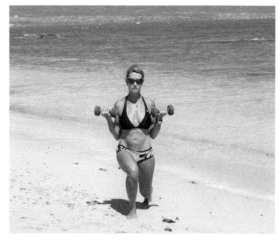

Exercise 5:
GET UP & GET DOWNS

All you need for these is a sturdy chair or bench. Good form is a must.

Begin by sitting down on the bench or chair with both feet out in front of you firmly placed on the ground with a 90 degree bend at the knee, shoulder width apart and with good posture. Be sure your toes are pointing forward. Try not lead with your head.

Start with your hands in front of you as you simply rise to a full standing position, driving up through your heel. *What is cheating on this move? By not returning to a full, seated position with all your weight on the bench, you are cheating yourself out a great exercise.*

Step up the tempo and go for it.

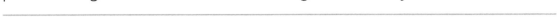

SUGGESTED EQUIPMENT
Workout bench, heavy chair, 8 pound medicine ball or dumbbell

SUGGESTED REPS/SETS/TIME
20-25 reps, 2-3 sets, or timed 1-2 minutes

PROGRESSION VARIABLES
Hold hands high above your head for the entire set or add an 8 pound medicine ball or dumbbell. Simply hold the weight in front of you at chest level. As you stand up press the weight out and forward. Return weight to chest as you sit back down.

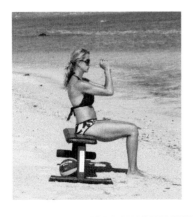
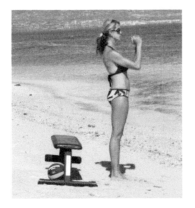
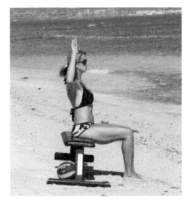

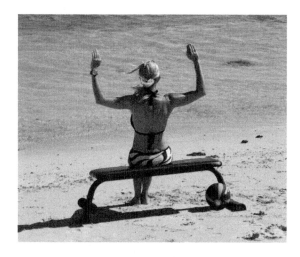 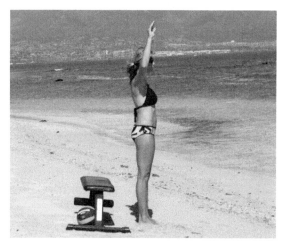

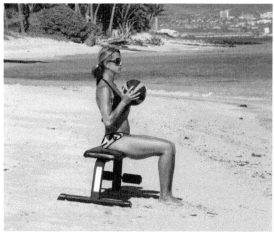 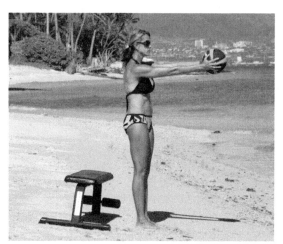

CIRCUIT TRAINING

Circuit training is one of *THE* most effective ways to increase your heart capacity. It keeps you moving, it's totally fun, and can be different every time. You can also include stand up paddling in your circuit.

Circuit training is one of the most time-efficient methods of cardio training and offers similar effects as traditional forms of cardio endurance training. Circuit training involves completing a variety of exercises with minimal rest. You will not get bored, which also helps you keep from plateauing in your overall training program.

This is a good time to bring out the heart rate monitor to track and record your efforts.

You can select exercises with or without weights as you create different stations with particular, preset goals. The trick is selecting the appropriate exercises that offer the best means of stimulation but are not too over the top or too difficult. You don't want to set yourself up to fail.

I suggest you keep your circuit training simple at first; you can move to more difficult and challenging exercises once you get the feel of it. First, know that you can perform circuit training within your current workout routine, make it exclusively a separate workout, or do both. You can make it your choice of cardio training for that session or let it be your standalone cardio choice for that day.

So for example, if your training day consists of your usual, active warm up, core work, balance work, and total body exercises, during the strength portion of your workout perform each following exercise at a faster tempo without any rest in between and you'll have done some circuit training. Or, instead of doing 2-3 sets of shoulders, chest, legs, biceps, etc., you can do one set of shoulders, then immediately follow with one set of chest, one set of legs, then biceps and triceps. Then, without rest, begin the second round in the same order at the same tempo.

It looks like this:

2-3 sets, 10-12 reps, no rest at a medium to fast tempo
Note: If you increase tempo, decrease weight.

1. Shoulders, 2-arm press
2. Back-Prone, 2-arm rows
3. Chest, push ups
4. Legs, squats
5. Biceps, 2-arm curls
6. Triceps, bench dips

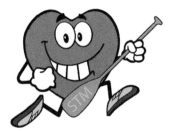

After you've completed your first set, you start at the top again and repeat. I saved the abs for last, as I always do with all of my suggested programs, for the simple reason that you need your abs to support you throughout your entire workout. Give them a break until the end and then crush them hard.

That's just one way to approach it.

Another example is to set up certain "cardio" producing exercise stations, say of 4-6 selected exercises. Include at least two of them to be in the "prone," or face down position, as your heart will be required to work 4 times harder this way. To avoid any dizziness, be careful when making your transitions from the ground back up to a standing position. You can also simply pick a high number of, say, 20-25 reps if you're using super light to no weights, and do 2-3 sets with no rest in between.

That might look like this:

Sample Circuit Station: 2-3 sets/circuits, 20-25 reps, no rest

1. Butt kicks
2. 5-8 pounds bicep curls
3. Mountain climbers on BOSU (prone position)
4. Ice skaters
5. 5-8 pounds weights tanding, bent over, 2 arm back rows (prone position)
6. Jumping jacks

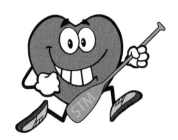

Check your heart rate, record your results.
Simple but fun! I promise you your heart rate will soar.

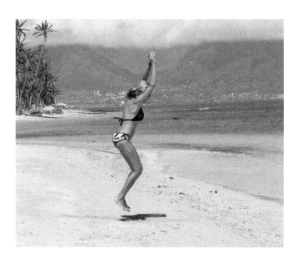 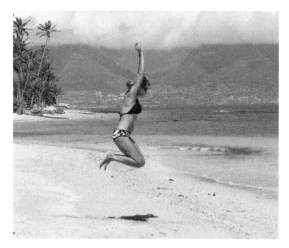

Exercise 1:
SAMPLE STAND UP PADDLE CIRCUIT: BOP STYLE

When we think of BOP we think of carnage. Not here. You can have that visual if it helps but you won't have any boards or other paddlers to dodge.

Most of you won't have access to a buoy but we can simply count strokes for the paddle portion. Make sure you're covering a short distance that's not too far from land, and that conditions are safe.

Keep it super simple and use your own body weight as a workout option, selecting exercises that keep you moving. You can also time yourself to max number of reps if you're wearing a watch.

On the beach I set up coconuts to zigzag around like threading the needle. I also use them as markers on the ground for other formations I need for other creative training tactics. You can use small cones, a sunscreen bottle, or slipper—whatever works. Just make it fun.

Sample SUP Water to Land Circuit: 2-3 sets/circuits, no rest

SUGGESTED EQUIPMENT
SUP board/paddle, coconuts, cones, or driftwood for markers, and medium-gauge tubing

SUGGESTED REPS/ROUNDS, SETS/CIRCUITS
20-25 reps, 2-3 sets, or timed 1-2 minutes. SUP board component: 50-75 strokes 3x per round/circuit

PROGRESSION VARIABLES
Paddle into wind, side chop, train in sand, add additional circuit

---

PROGRESSION 1

4 Point Side Shuffles: One Round

Set coconuts or cones or any other object 3-5 feet apart in a straight line. Start at the first cone and quickly shuffle to the right, moving to cone two. Touch cone with right hand and then shuffle back to cone one, touching with left hand. Then shuffle fast all the way to cone three, touching it with your right hand and then shuffle back to cone one, and the finally shuffle to cone four and all the way back to cone number one. In sand this is exciting!

NO REST

PROGRESSION 2

Standing Tube Bicep Curls: 15-20 fast.

Stand on tubing with two feet, holding a handle in each hand. Bend your knees and stand with chest out and shoulders back and perform the bicep curls. To increase difficulty spread feet apart.

NO REST

PROGRESSION 3

Paddle

Grab your board and hit the water. Run if you want to go BOP style; hop up and go. Keep your head clear and focused and remember that in your final round or count of 50-75 strokes you will go all out. So start with a fast cadence and keep counting in whatever increments you need to reach your target number. On your second effort, hard pivot turn or turn and head back with your final count of 50-75 strokes. Don't forget to take off your leash before jumping off the board. RUN back to next station.

NO REST

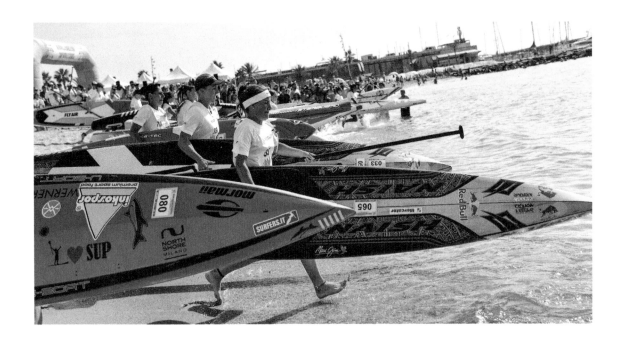

PROGRESSION 4

Alternating Split Lunges with Hands Behind Head: 15-20

Start with a split wide stance keeping your knee directly over your foot. Push off the feet at the same time and switch to bring the other leg into a lunge and land softly. With your hands behind your head you will have to balance more.

NO REST

PROGRESSION 5

Knee Bent or Standard Push ups: 15-20

Perform a knee bent push up or standard push up at a fast tempo. Stand up slowly at a count to three.

Repeat this entire circuit 2-3 more times. Drink plenty of fluids and fuel properly.

Check your heart rate; record your results.

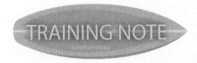
There are many ways you can perform your own circuit training. This is a small sample.

Next we talk about a more explosive way to bring your heart rate up and that's called plyometric training.

PLYOMETRICS

Here is where you shock the system—the heart system, that is. Now that you have some new total body moves and you've also discovered ways to add circuit training to your cardio training, your body is semi-used to handling a bit more total body stress. I'm going to introduce to you another form of training—called plyometrics—that's been around forever.

It is a really explosive method of training and is designed to generate high levels of power. In doing so it also can really increase your heart capacity to achieve high levels of SUP performance.

Although our focus here is to increase your heart capacity these types of exercise are also used to increase speed and endurance. This is a bonus. Because we are paddlers and need to strengthen our upper and lower body I will include both.

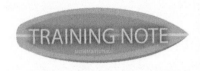

Because plyometric training involves jumping and bounding, one should have a good level of fitness and not exhibit any major joint or muscle injury when attempting these exercises. You also may want to adjust the number of reps and sets until your body and heart adapts.

I also suggest a proper warm up of active stretching, or a light 3 minute jog, ten jumping jacks and a few squats to prepare your body. You will also be burning a higher amount of calories and could also lose body fluids at a higher rate so be well prepared to hydrate before during and after. You should also apply a nice cool down session as well.

FIVE PLYOMETRIC EXERCISES

Exercise 1:
DOUBLE BURPEES WITH A PUSH UP

These are also known as squat thrusts. Double your fun with the double burpees. Everyone is doing it! You might taste your lunch while doing these so be careful. Burpees basically combine a squat, push up, and vertical leap. These are TOUGH.

Similar to the standard burpee, but you'll do two leg kick outs behind you and two jumps up. For some reason I like these better than the standard burpees.

Begin by standing up tall with your feet about shoulder width apart. Lower yourself into a squat position with hands on the floor then kick out behind you fast. You should now be in a push up position. Perform a push up. As fast as possible thrust your feet forward again towards your hands and kick out again behind you.

Immediately jump up into the air with your hands high above you and, with a soft landing, jump up again. Repeat.

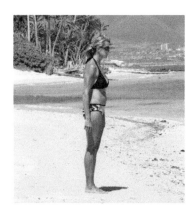
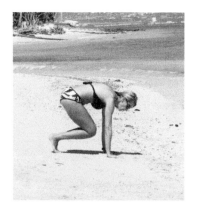
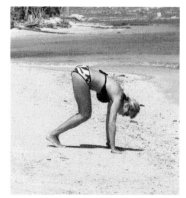

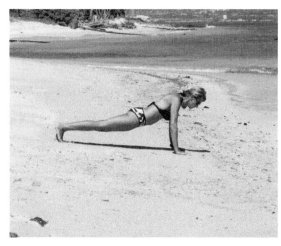
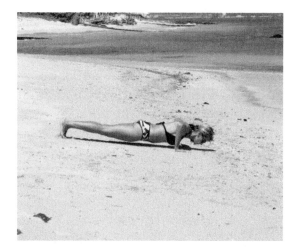

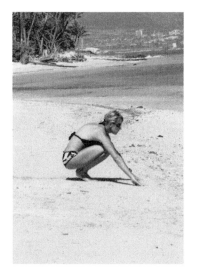
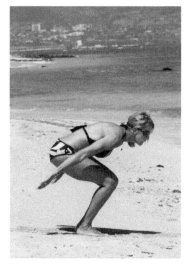
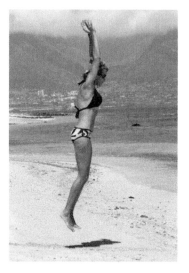

Exercise 2:
FRONT BOX JUMPS

While these will turn on your legs for sure, the goal here is to increase your heart rate.

SUGGESTED EQUIPMENT
Sturdy square platform 6-36 inches high

SUGGESTED REPS/SETS/TIME
12-15 reps, 2-3 sets

PROGRESSION VARIABLES
You can either increase box height or add weight via weighted vest, barbell or dumbbells to increase the difficulty.
***You may also attempt by using only one leg, but this is for the most advanced.

Stand directly in front of platform. Get into a squat position with your feet about shoulder-width apart. Squat and jump up with an explosive motion that uses your entire body, including your arms. Land softy on the box on the balls of your feet. Step down or hop down. Land softly, assume good form, and repeat.

Side story: In 2009 I broke my left leg and both ankles and spent 3 months in a wheelchair. My legs turned to mush and this box has been my bugaboo ever since. When I stand there I have a conversation with it and tell it, "I conquer you now." Hope that helps!

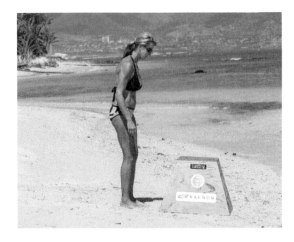
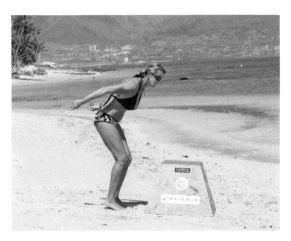

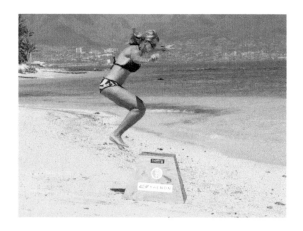 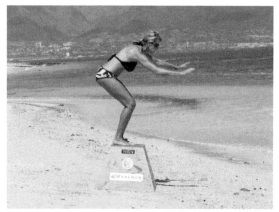

Exercise 3:
SCISSOR JUMPS

These are one of my favorites. The key is to find a rhythm and land softly.

SUGGESTED EQUIPMENT
None

SUGGESTED REPS/SETS/TIME
20-25, reps, 2-3 sets, timed 1-2 minutes

PROGRESSION VARIABLES
Increase tempo and keep reaching higher as you jump

Get into a standard lunge position, keeping your back straight and your knees and toes forward. Squat down and explode up, switching leg positions in mid-air. Land softly and immediately transition to your next jump. Perform the same movement, switching your leg position each time.

Exercise 4:
CONTINUOUS BROAD JUMPS

These are fun and all you need is a big open space. These are also known as bounding jumps. Again, your legs are the driving force but your arms are also what help you move forward.

SUGGESTED EQUIPMENT
Large open space, grass or track, sand

SUGGESTED REPS/SETS/TIME
12-15 reps, 2-3 sets

PROGRESSION VARIABLES
Increase tempo, change surface from flat to sand. (Note) These are very difficult in sand.

Facing an open space, begin in a squat position with your feet shoulder-width apart. Squat down deep and, with the use of your arms, explode up, and forward. Land softly on the ground and immediately transition into your next rep.

Exercise 5:
SKATERS WITH A JUMP

This time we move in a lateral direction. These use the entire body with a focus, however, on a single leg at a time, which can also help with balance. You'll be thrusting your body into the air, requiring a soft, stabilizing landing on each leg.

SUGGESTED EQUIPMENT
Studio floor, grass or track, sand

SUGGESTED REPS/SETS/TIME
20-25 reps, 2-3 sets, timed 1-2 minutes

PROGRESSION VARIABLES
Increase tempo, change surface from flat to sand. (Note) These are very difficult in sand. Add weight with a medicine ball.

Get into a squat position with your feet close together and the majority of your weight on your right leg. Push off your right leg to the opposite side. Land softly on your left leg and move your right leg behind like you would while ice skating. Repeat on your left leg. That's one rep.

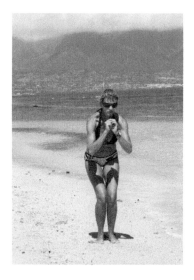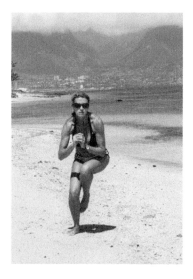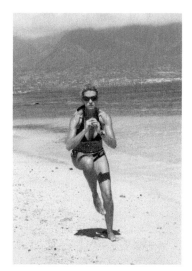

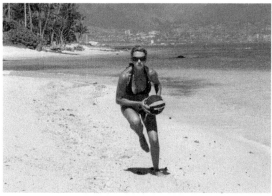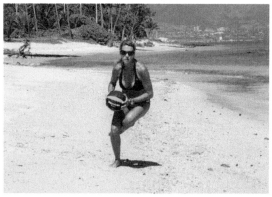

This concludes the plyometric training. You have now learned that there are many different ways to stimulate your heart and increase your heart capacity.

SAMPLE CARDIO PROGRAMS

While there are many exercises, variables, and methods to choose from while designing your own cardio program, I'd like to give you a few samples and options of programs that you might enjoy. If anything, it will get you thinking of ways to incorporate cardio training as you become a stronger paddler.

Below I give you five sample cardio programs. You can also add one these programs to your current strength training regime as your cardio component. You can pick one program to try one day and then another for the following session. Feel free to substitute and modify any exercises you need in order to assure your success and safety.

These programs are going to be focusing on three different energy systems during your workouts: aerobic, anaerobic and alactate power:

- Aerobic (70-75% of your max HR)
- Anaerobic (80-85% of your max HR)
- Alactate Power (90-100% max HR)

Refer to reference section below for more information.

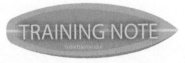

As with any workout you begin, complete a 2-3 minute warm up. A warm up could include a light jog, jumping jacks, active stretching, simple half squats, or any movements that provide full body stimulation.

I would also incorporate 2-3 core exercises from Chapter 2 before your begin your program of choice. Just do one of these per day, not all five. A proper cool down is also important for a successful session.

Remember, have fun, simple is best, hydrate and fuel properly, and I'll see you at the finish line.

Paddle Pump One
Combines a combination of **Plyometrics** and **light weights** and one dynamic exercise with paddling in mind.

You will notice that I selected two exercises that place your body in the prone position as that will increase your heart output by 4 times. I also selected exercises with every body part in mind.

Paddle Pump One				NO REST
Exercise	Reps	Sets	Tempo	Notes
Scissor Jumps	20-25	2-3	Fast	Soft landing, use arms
Mountain Climbers	20-25	2-3	Fast	BOSU/ground, keeps abs drawn in
Standing Bicep Curls	20-25	2-3	Fast	3-10pounds, chest out, bend knees
Push ups	20-25	2-3	Fast	Knee bent or split set
TRX Rip Trainer Paddling Strokes	1 min R&L	2-3	Fast	You can split 30s with short or longer strokes, dig in

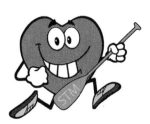 Check your heart rate, record your results.

Paddle Pump Two

Consists of the total body exercises mentioned early in this chapter.

Paddle Pump Two				NO REST
Exercise	Reps	Sets	Tempo	Notes
Kettle Bell Swings	15-20	2-3	Moderate	Good posture, squeeze glutes
Squat to Shoulder Press	15-20	2-3	Moderate	Smooth and controlled, add weight as desired
Mountain Climbers	15-20	2-3	Moderate	BOSU, floor. Indoboard plus Gigante Cushion
Split Lunge Two Arm Bicep Curl	15-20	2-3	Moderate	Watch lunge form, add weight as desired

Check your heart rate, record your results

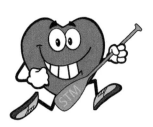

Paddle Pump Three

Includes **paddling, Plyometrics, agility**, courage and guts.

Paddle Pump Three				NO REST
Exercise	Reps	Sets	Tempo	Notes
BOSU Agility Drill	25	2-3	Fast	Up and over side to side
SUP Paddle Sprints	50-75 strokes x3 per set	2-3	Fast Super Fast	Complete 2 rounds, pivot turn paddle hard back to shore
BOSU 1 Arm/ alternating Push ups	10/10	2-3	Moderate	Complete 10 with one hand on top. Knee bent or standard
Skaters with A Jump	25	2-3	Moderate	Don't forget the jump, land softly and stabilize

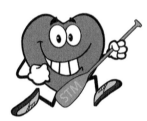 Check your heart rate, record your results.

Paddle Pump Four

This is more of a **traditional form of circuit training** that includes all muscle groups. You can use the weight amount you would normally, allowing this to qualify as a strength training session as well as cardio. You could also round off this session with a 15 minute spin bike session or run outside.

Paddle Pump Four				NO REST
Exercise	Reps	Sets	Tempo	Notes
Shoulders-Tube Chops	10-12	2-3	Moderate	Floor, progress to unstable
Chest Pec Flys	10-12	2-3	Moderate	Stability ball bridge position
Back 1 Arm Lawnmower	10-12	2-3	Moderate	Head neutral, draw in abs
Legs Hamstring Curls	10-12	2-3	Moderate	Perform on stability ball
Biceps – Seated 2 arm	10-12	2-3	Moderate	Two legs to unstable platform
Triceps- Tube Presses	10-12	2-3	Moderate	Good posture, 2 second hold
**Abs last Chest Lifts DO LAST AT END	100-150	2-3	Moderate	Support neck, back flat, elbows flat, look behind you, lift, breathe

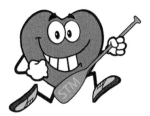 Check your heart rate, record your results.

Paddle Pump Five

This program is all **Plyometrics** and if you're not quite ready for this just modify it if you need to. This program does primarily focus on the legs, so be aware.

Paddle Pump Five				NO REST
Exercise	**Reps**	**Sets**	**Tempo**	**Notes**
Continuous Broad Jumps	10	2-3	Fast	Thrust forward with arms for momentum, don't stop
Double Burpees	10	2-3	Moderate/ Fast	Watch your form, don't get sloppy
Skaters with A Jump	10	2-3	Moderate	Thrust upward with arms, land softly stabilize, repeat
Front Box Jump	10	2-3	Moderate	Thrust upward with arms, land with two feet on box

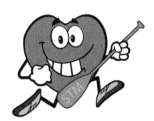 Check your heart rate, record your results.

In addition to the exercises and approaches I've mentioned above there so are many ways you can add cardio to current paddling training routine. Walking is great, so is performing interval sprints. Running, mountain or road cycling, and swimming are also great choices.

I have lots of clients and friends who are competitive paddlers and the swimmers tend to have tremendous lung capacity. And just as a reminder, swimming one mile, which is not that easy, is equivalent to running four miles.

Maybe your local gym offers what are called fusion fit classes or other types of aerobic classes. Tennis is amazing and great for leg strengthening too.

Now that you've stepped up your heart game to achieve your **SUPreme state of performance paddling**, your stroke and cadence will be stronger and faster as well. If you find yourself getting hung up on technical paddling issues, it may be time for a professional coaching session. I'm always here to help.

This concludes this chapter on cardio training to increase your stand up paddling performance. I imagine that, for some of you, these exercises may have been familiar and for others maybe they were new. Either way by incorporating some of my programs or combining a few different routines and approaches to your current one your performance should now be on the rise.

In Chapter 7, called The Mental Part, it's time to get your head into your paddling and discover ways in which you can get into a good mental state to help you perform at your best. Check it out.

REFERENCE TERMS:

Aerobic: Aerobic (70-75% of your max HR) – a level of work you can continue for an extended period of time (more than 3 minutes) and using oxygen to help provide the calorie/fat burn for energy.

Anaerobic: Anaerobic (80-85% of your max HR) – a level of work where lactic acid builds up faster than your body can remove it. You use more stored glycogen than fat at this intensity—but you also burn more calories overall than the aerobic energy system. This level of work keeps your body burning more calories after exercise is done as well (post paddle calorie burn—PPCB).

Anaerobic threshold (AT): is the point at which the body can no longer produce enough energy for the muscles with normal oxygen intake. As a result, it begins to produce higher levels of lactic acid than can be removed from the body. So therefore, your main goal is to increase your anaerobic threshold.

Alactate power: (90-100% max HR) – You can only manage this level of exercise for periods of up to 12 seconds. Burns a lot of calories and also has high PECB.

Bonk: Also referred to as hitting the wall, describes a condition caused by the depletion of glycogen stores in the liver and muscles, which manifests itself by sudden fatigue and loss of energy. The condition can usually be avoided by making sure that glycogen levels are high when the exercise begins, maintaining glucose levels during exercise by eating or drinking carbohydrate-rich substances, or by reducing exercise intensity.

Heart rate (HR): The rate with which the heart pumps is referred to as the heart rate. The heart rate of the typical person is roughly 70-80 beats per min (bpm). A very fit person's resting heart rate may be 40-60 bpm.

Interval training: Combines short bursts of all out speed followed by a slower recovery phase then repeated over the course of a pre-determined length of time, and is often repeated at regular intervals. It usually last from 15 seconds to sometimes 30 seconds. For example, you could jog for 30 minutes and then sprint for 15 seconds, return to a jog and then repeat this every five minutes.

Max heart rate: The highest heart rate that can be attained by an individual in strenuous activity, varying with fitness and, in adults, inversely with age. A "rule-of-thumb" formula for the predicted maximum is 220 – your age. If you are more fit you can use the formula of 205 – age.

Perceived level of exertion: Also known as RPE or "Rate of Perceived Exertion" **(Refer to my graph above)**, it is a way of measuring physical activity intensity level and the feelings you may feel in relation to strain, stress and/or discomfort, and state of breathing during exercise of any kind. How hard you are working or your RPE, can then be measured on a number scale. Perceived exertion is how hard you feel like your body is working. For example the number 1-2 is no work to light work, and 10 would be extremely intense or max.

Recovery heart rate: Recovery heart rate is your heart's ability to return to a normal rate after an activity within a specific amount of time. In general, a faster heart rate (HR) recovery (HR slowing down) from an activity is an indication of an improved fitness level.

Resting heart rate: Simply means your rate when you're at rest. Typically the normal resting heart rate for adults ranges from 60 to 100 beats per minute. Generally, a lower heart rate at rest implies more efficient heart function and better cardiovascular fitness. For example, a well-trained paddler might have a normal resting heart rate closer to 40 beats a minute. For men the average resting heart rate is usually between 70 and 72 beats per minute, and for women it is usually between 78 and 82 bpm.

VO2 Max: VO2Max refers to the maximum amount of oxygen that an individual can utilize during intense or maximal exercise. It is measured as "milliliters of oxygen used in one minute per kilogram of body weight."

Reference for Footnote: Target Heart Rate Table from *Heart.Org Sportsmedicine.About.com*

Dr. Hirofumi Tanaka, PhD WebMd.

CHAPTER 7
The Mental Part

- Thinking like A SUP athlete and training for greatness.
- What is visualization training and how it can it increase your paddling performance?
- What it means to be mentally fit for SUP: A special excerpt from Annabel Anderson after her 2015 M20 win.
- Paddling "in the Zone": What it means and how to get there.
- What are the defining characteristics of paddler able to get in the zone?
- Removing barriers and obstacles to clear your path for SUP success.

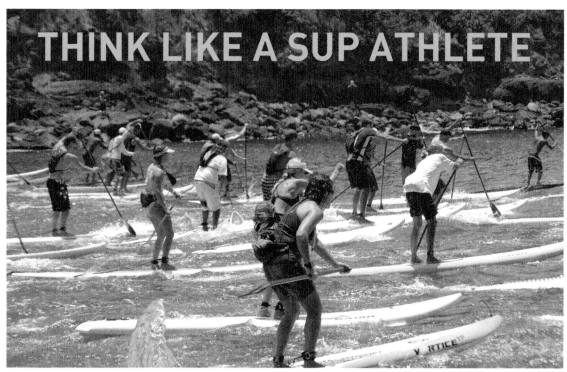

THINK LIKE A SUP ATHLETE

photo by Casey Fukua

TIPS AND PRACTICES ON HOW TO STRENGTHEN YOUR MENTAL GAME FOR SUP

It's a known scientific fact that if you look at and focus on the muscle you are training it will respond, adapt, and perform to your expectations. I'm hoping that by the time you finish reading this chapter you will stand at the water's edge with board and paddle and respond to the changes and new *growth* in your mind and body. The mind is a powerful tool, but that's just the beginning of what you're going to learn in this chapter.

While goals such as winning a race, not missing one training day, eating healthier, and so forth, are important, how about thinking a bit more long-term? Have you heard of the post-SUP event blues? Maybe you've had a particular feeling after you've trained hard for a big event. You end up doing pretty well, and then, after all the Facebook hoopla and ra ra, you feel kind of empty and deflated? Then you look around, shrug your shoulders, and seek what's "next?" Sound familiar?

I've had that feeling a few times, where I feel temporarily bummed—not knowing what to do with myself. After a big race I'm not as disciplined with training and, while not all the wheels fall off the wagon, I tend to ease up and slack off for a week or two. I eat what I want maybe have a glass of wine. Rest and recovery are important but mentally I kind of feel, hmmm, okay. . . gee. "The thrill is gone" kind of thing. I want that lovin' feeling back of having something to train for.

How about this time around as you approach your SUP performance training you maybe put the word "growth" into your brain? Yes, it's a bit more than most commitment phobics can handle, but if you put your best stroke forward time and time again and continue to learn even from your past losses, current wins, and maybe unexpected detours, you'll feel even a bigger reward as you paddle through life. Make sense?

You and I are in this book for the distance, not just the sprint across the lake. Focus on the now and savor it. Taste your victories and embrace your losses as part of the journey to make you a more mentally fit paddler.

What kind of paddler do you "see" when you think of yourself? Do you see a strong, fire-breathing dragon of a SUP racer, or do you see a happy go lucky golden retriever content just to tootle along and have fun? There is no right answer as long as you are happy with what you see and you are having fun.

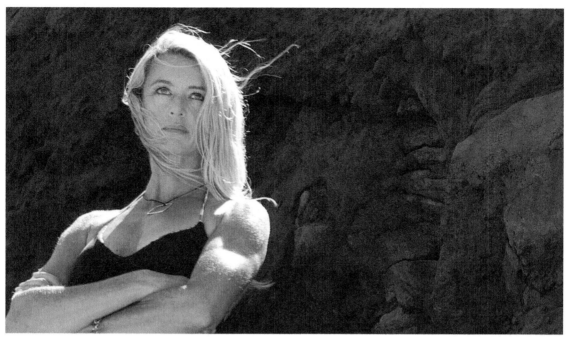

photo by Tracy Leboe

Are there times on race day when you second-guess your strength, confidence, or paddling technique? Are you nervous about paddling with people that may be better than you and you don't feel you can keep up? Do you ever feel emotionally defeated and down on yourself when you don't finish well? Or are you able to take inventory, acknowledge what you can do better, shake it off, and keep doing your best?

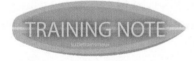

At this very moment, I want you now to "see" yourself as a SUP athlete. You must think, speak, eat, train, and paddle like a SUP athlete if you want to be a stronger stand up paddler. I wanted to say walk and talk, but I'm not sure how a paddler walks?

You've heard the saying: "If you're going to talk the talk, you've got to walk the walk."

What I say to that is "If you're going to paddle like you mean it, you'd better mean it and paddle."

I have a story about myself that may come as a surprise to some of you. You see, all my life I enjoyed a lot of sports. And you might think, "Well, she's a trainer and lives on Maui so she must be a good athlete. Look what she does for a living and where she lives?" I have to work very hard at changing gears from trainer to athlete, myself. It just doesn't happen. Trainers rarely have time to train themselves.

As a matter of fact I've never really seen myself as an athlete even though at young age I was a sponsored dirt bike racer and loved the speed. Even though I raced a bit and finished my last race at the famous Hangtown track, I was riding because I loved motorcycles and the thrill of going fast. I just happened to be decent, I guess. I didn't compare myself to the other kids. I just admired them and did my own thing.

Several years later, at the age of 17, I traded dirt for water and caught the windsurfing bug. I really got into it and sailed my brains out until I literally couldn't walk, got banged up pretty hard from head to toe and discovered later I had no off switch in my brain. That left me with many serious injuries then and down the road, some of which still affect me.

Training? I didn't know what training was. I just went out and did it. I ate at McDonalds because it was good and it was cheap. Horrible. I do remember that I could curl a 15 pound dumbbell when I was 16, so I thought that was cool and it probably came in handy. But a regular training regime for me did not exist. I played tennis now and then and would go to the park and run, but never with a planned intention.

I entered a few windsurf races in the Bay Area and once made the front page of the Sacramento Bee. I had a couple of great sponsors to help me out but nothing too serious. It was so mellow then. One thing for sure is I always had Maui on my mind and started to visualize living here. How I got here is another story for another book. Please stay tuned for that one; it's halfway done.

So now I get to say, "If I only knew then what I know now." Would I have been a stronger, smarter, athlete? I would have to assume "yes" to all.

Had I seen and thought of myself as an athlete back then, maybe I would have sailed smarter, eaten healthier, ridden my dirt bike with my brain and have avoided some serious, long-term injuries. But no, I hacked away at my non-smart, non-thinking athlete life. I was young and unbreakable.

Fast forward. I moved to Maui, changing my former career and life plan to follow my passions to help and serve others. I got into SUP in late 2008 and, well, you know the rest of the story.

On July 27th, 2014 when I was in the middle of Kai'wi" channel somewhere between Molokai and Oahu, I was very confident I would finish the M2O race. It wasn't, however, until I got to the finish that I said to myself, with a big smile, *"Suzie, you are officially an athlete."* I was pretty proud of myself and that left a lifelong imprint that I will never forget. It was a real confidence booster.

Having my cheering squad and coach Jeremy Riggs on the boat and feeling unstoppable—in the zone—was life changing. I simply can't describe it. To see a video of our journey and to read more about what it was like crossing the channel visit my website: *http://bit.ly/1hAerHM*

In this chapter I'll talk about what it's like being in the proverbial "zone" and how to achieve a state of consciousness and awareness to help you get there.

I'll help you discover ways to help you remove physical and mental barriers that may be preventing you from performing at your absolute best in SUP.

To help you achieve the mental strength and endurance that you need to perform your best SUP possible, I'll offer effective tips and best practices to strengthen your mental muscle.

This leads me to our first topic: the power of the mind to receive certain suggestive thoughts and visuals of how we see ourselves navigate in life and in SUP.

THINKING LIKE A SUP ATHLETE

If a thought is defined as "an idea or opinion produced by thinking or occurring suddenly in the mind," if we produce the *thought* that we are SUP athletes and have the *opinion or idea* that we are, then we *are* SUP athletes.

To be an amazing SUP athlete takes hard work, dedication, maybe a little talent, and lots and lots of training. The one component people seem to overlook is the mental part or the emotional and psychological work that must also be done to achieve such a status.

Do you remember how it felt to enter your first SUP race or event? Whether it was serious or not, you couldn't help to feel a little giddy and probably nervous too.

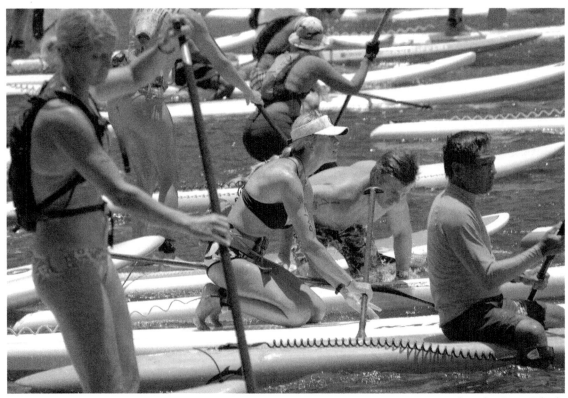

photo by Casey Fukuda

Here's the snapshot: Your division is next. You're standing there with your board and paddle getting ready to walk to the water's edge. You do a final check: hydration pack, sunscreen, visor or hat, leash, rash guard—check, check, check, check.

You look to the left at all the other paddlers and scan to the right, seeing more paddlers looking pretty serious. You say to yourself, "Wow, gulp; these guys look like real SUP athletes. What the hell am I doing here? I'm probably going to finish last." When you think these things are you thinking like a SUP athlete?

No.

You could say, "It's show time. I'm freak'n gonna paddle my heart out and crush it. I feel great and I'm ready because I am a fierce competitor. I am a SUP athlete."

That is thinking like a SUP athlete.

It doesn't matter what brand of board you paddle, how many followers you have on Instagram or the color of the rash guard you wear, it's how you think about and see yourself that really matters.

Having a healthy self-image as a confident and competent SUP athlete is a good thing. It's not okay to be cocky and a braggart but if you have high levels of confidence your paddling skill level will be higher as well.

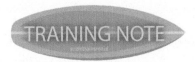 *Thinking confidently as a SUP athlete reflects or mirrors the desired result.*

Anticipate success by being self-confident. Prepare, physically and emotionally. These are great character traits to build upon that will enhance your SUP performance skills and produce winning outcomes.

If winning more SUP races is your goal, prepare your mind to win and see yourself on the podium. Think and say to yourself, "I am a SUP athlete and a winner." If simply becoming more efficient at downwind paddling is your goal, prepare a new mind shift of seeing yourself catching every bump and glide. Think and say to yourself, "I am a good downwind paddler catching lots of bumps and glides."

Remember: confidence often mirrors the skills you wish to achieve. You are a SUP athlete.

HOW VISUALIZATION TRAINING CAN INCREASE YOUR SUP PERFORMANCE

One day after a morning session on the north shore here on Maui, my dear friend, mentor, and client Wendall DeVera walked over to my truck for a little talk story. I shared with him that I'm writing this book and having so much fun learning and exploring all about the power of the mind and visualization training. (Just a side note, he's an amazing canoe paddler and Tai Chi instructor with years and years of experience. He is also owner of TriPaddle.)

His eyes lit up as we got to talking more about how he sees and feels himself paddling across the water during his Tai Chi practices. He said to me, "Suzie you must first paddle slow to paddle fast." I stopped all my thoughts and thought, wow that is so true.

He began to demonstrate, reaching his arms forward, his eyes almost in a trancelike state. He reached forward with his bottom shoulder, turning his chest towards me. He closed his eyes and continued this stroke-like motion and said, "See, the slower you go the more efficient you become." Something so simple is absolutely so true. I remember Dave Kalama talking about this too.

He had originally hired me to help make him faster while he was seated in his boat. I thought, "Okay, we can find cool ways to train his core and hips so he can feel and transfer that to his boat." I really enjoyed each and every session. He would come so prepared and was very disciplined. He paid attention to my every cue. I was so impressed with the thoughtful execution of every repetition.

He went on to share that as he teaches Tai Chi, he helps people learn that everything comes from the ground up. So while we were training his visual was the ocean being the ground and the boat was the connection to his hips, his core, his shoulders and his mind. It was all very cool.

We can apply the same theory or suggestion to SUP. Every stroke comes from the surface of the water to our brain, then through our board to our hips, to our core, obliques, the shoulders, and then to the paddle.

Visualization training is not a new concept. It is actually a powerful training tool used by the best in the world. Sports psychologists, trainers, and coaches alike also refer to it as guided imagery, meditation, mental rehearsal, and a few other things.

Four years ago I wrote an article called: *What You See Is How You Perform: Increase Your SUP, Surf, Dirt biking, or Any Sports Performance with Visualization Training*

The article starts like this: See the finish line, the crowd cheering you on the last buoy turn, the last surf heat before the horn, the last lap of your mountain bike or dirt bike race and see *your* personal victory! Okay, now adjust the speed and tempo, add a little more weight to the bar, do a few more balance tricks, and turn up the music.

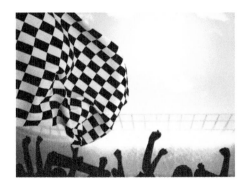

To read the rest of the article, visit my website: *http://bit.ly/1NOgWnr*

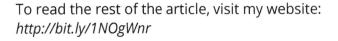

Other stimuli you can imagine—other than an image or visual—could include elements of how you feel, what you hear, or even what you taste when you are successful. The more vivid you can paint the picture or visuals of your outcome to include your feeling—and even tastes—the more positive your performance will be.

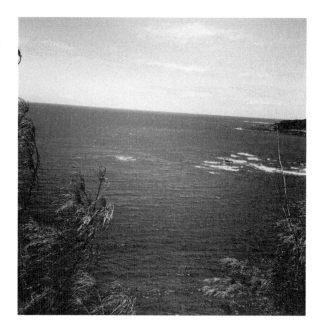

I like to have this particular visual of Maliko Gulch. I like to see the white caps building in my mind and smell the salt air. I can feel the winds swirling on my face then on my back as I exit. I like to look at the tall, steep cliffs before I enter the magic blue carpet. This really helps me focus in my training.

For example you may remember what it felt like to really push your body during a difficult SUP race—crossing that finish line and feeling really good about that day. You may also dream of having those feelings—the surging feelings of adrenaline crossing that finish line, seeing and hearing your friends cheer you on, the smell of the ocean, and maybe the taste of sweat dripping down your forehead. Sounds like a great race to me!

Here is a great shot of my awesome client Bo Forster completing her first downwind race at the Olukai Ho'olaule'a this year. It was an 8 mile surfing race for sure. I was so proud of her. What a rewarding day as a coach.

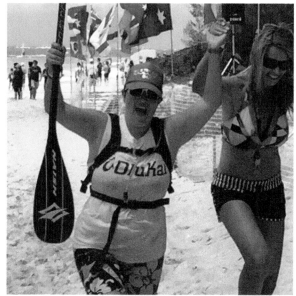

That's what I'm talking about here. Try to capture and save those vivid, particular feelings—those visuals, those smells and sounds. In addition to being motivational, they are also great memories that remain with you forever.

Now think of your mind as a huge database recalling files and files of images of you winning the race or reaching your training goal. Add all of those feelings and smells and sounds and tastes.

Come race day your subconscious retrieves those winning images and feelings that allow your mind and body to shape and make that outcome true. Your confidence will soar and hopefully you'll do very well.

You can also apply these practices to your training in the gym and on the water. I do it all the time. I have goals for each training session, so before I begin a paddling session or lift some weights, I've already recalled some amazing images from past races that help me get motivated before I train.

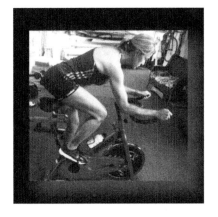

Here are a few things I do before a typical gym training session. I prepare my music and water. I write down the date and time in my training journal before I start. I put on my heart rate monitor, and all the while, I'm seeing visuals in my head of the outcome of a race coming up or how well I want to do on my next Maliko downwinder with the guys.

After a warm up, I'm on my spin bike, and I get into a nice steady rhythm with legs and breath before I do an interval sprint. I see myself walking to the water's edge and putting my board in the water. Then I visualize myself attaching my leash, taking a few practice strokes and looking out to scan the water and reefs breaking to my right.

As the music begins to get a little faster I'm pedaling faster. I see myself paddling a bit harder getting out of Maliko Gulch. I look upwind at all of the whitecaps that are building then BOOM, the music tempo switches to high gear with some heavy metal song blasting, and so do I. The scene in my head is me turning left then down the ocean to begin the most amazing downwinder ever. Gee! I was getting super excited as I was typing, getting this visual going in my head.

I visualize paddling, my mouth starting to get a bit dry because I expended a bit of energy getting out against the side swell and now it's game time. I'm taking a sip from my CamelBak and scanning and on the hunt for the best and biggest trough to launch me on a 100 yard glide. Wow, thinking of this makes me want to go right now! Okay, back to you.

I'm sure you get the idea. Having the visuals of yourself paddling at higher levels in skill, speed, and endurance will help you shape a positive outcome for yourself.

I will be sharing more a bit later in this chapter and talking about the other side of visualizing a positive outcome. It's also important to learn how to manage circumstances when the outcomes aren't so good. I'll discuss how you can develop tools to visualize yourself getting out of a bad situation calmly and turning it around to a positive or better one.

WHAT DOES IT MEAN TO BE MENTALLY FIT FOR STAND UP PADDLING: SPECIAL EXCERPT FROM ANNABEL ANDERSON AFTER HER 2015 M20 WIN

This has been an unusual year in Hawaii as, normally, the strong trade winds grace our island chain making for exciting channel races. These races, such as the prestigious Molokai to Oahu race, are usually wild adventures. Instead, this year the winds decided to take a break, testing the best of the best to an open ocean endurance, long paddling marathon, with high heat and humidity. A gigantic swell awaited the paddlers at the finish, putting boats and racers in serious situations.

Annabel Anderson, who decided not long before the race to give it a go, did what no woman has done and crushed the event by placing second overall on a stock 14ft board. Congrats again Annabel!

I had the chance to catch up with her a day after the race and we chatted for a couple of hours. I'm always intrigued with her insights and ability to break down and put to words how she does so well. Not only is she extremely physically fit but her mind is, too. She's a great writer so I was super stoked when she agreed to share some of her smarts with us for my book. She writes:

"Being 'mentally fit' for any kind of performance (be it work, school, sporting or otherwise) requires the mental, physical and emotional to all be in balance. I call it the triangle of equilibrium. If one is out, none of them are balanced. To produce a performance of your ultimate potential you need all three elements to be in balance.

Realistically, you may only ever truly be 'in the zone' a handful of times throughout your career. Most of us will struggle to attain mental, physical and emotional equilibrium simply due to the daily stresses of life.

Knowing this, one of the most important things you can do is to be in tune with your 'triangle of equilibrium' and work on a tool kit of skills to enable you to flip the 'equilibrium' switch even when things are out of balance. This only comes with time and practice. You have to know/work out how to trigger the switch to turn on your emotional and mental switches even in times of crises. If you don't have the mental and emotional, you will never be able to pull from your true physical capabilities to capitalize on the work and training you have put in (i.e. you have a relationship breakup leading into a major event, a close friend of family member passes away, all of your gear get lost by an airline or the conditions are not what you are comfortable in etc.).

Don't be afraid when things are out of whack. If you have trained yourself to bring yourself back to equilibrium, you'll be fine. Some people's best performances have happened when everything has gone wrong. But if you don't practice or develop a tool kit, you can't expect it to happen automatically."

Such a great take on how she mentally performs and prepares for her paddling success.

PADDLING IN THE ZONE: WHAT IT'S LIKE AND HOW TO GET THERE

I've heard many great athletes who say that when they're slipping into this state of greatness it feels as if time stands still, the water parts, and they're gliding across a magic carpet. You hear nothing. You see nothing. You just go. That is just one description of being in "the zone." Have you ever experienced something like this during a SUP race or while training?

Just the other day one of my clients who is a former skateboard pro, loves to trek on his motorcycle for hundreds of miles across the mainland, loves to paddle surf, and lives his life in the high RPM zone; said to me:

"When your mind is right is when you can do the most damage."

Wow. I stopped the medicine ball almost in mid air and thought, "That is so damn true." Good one Sidney and thank you.

The zone has also been referred to as the "flow" and/or "doing without doing." This is where all of the hard work, discipline, sacrifice, and hours (or years) of training seem to symbiotically line up and presents you with a moment in time when you become an unstoppable force, paddling in a way that can be descried as effortless.

Here is Kody Kerbox "in the zone" in Tahiti 2015

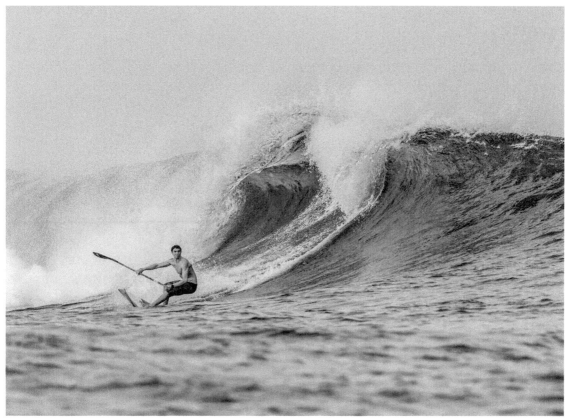

photo by Andrew Welker

Immediately after this sensation of total and complete focused absorption, some people break out in tears of joy, or, if they have been in this zone-like state for hours or days at a time, they may have completely passed out from forgetting to eat, sleep, and hydrate.

Paddling in the zone can happen often if you're well-trained and tuned in. There are also certain personality traits that tend to be pre-formatted in the minds of athletes who can often reach the zone. I'll touch on this a bit later.

If you have yet to experience it, don't panic or over think it. At this point you are more aware of what being in the zone may feel like. You could have already experienced it or your time could be coming soon. You will usually know when it happens but you may have no memory as to *how* it happened, but you loved it, or, I guarantee you will love it.

Being in the zone can have its own meaning to you, as well. Once you get connected to it and have been there, you may have already or will learn how to develop an ability to get there or build your way, which will be there for you to draw on when you need it at your next SUP race.

Some claim they can control it and others say it just happens. Being able to control it and turn it on and off when you need to is the ultimate goal. But is that really possible? What do you think?

Here's a cool quote that I got from **Jeremy Riggs** about how he experiences the zone. He writes,

"When I'm in the zone I feel like a super power out of my dreams is becoming real. When I'm tapped into the energy in that environment, I feel like I've become a part of nature. Nature's energy is flowing through me and I feel an amazing sense of freedom and belongingness. Every time it happens I can't believe it's happening. When it's over, I can't believe what just happened. It is such an amazing experience that I have made it my goal to help other people experience it for themselves."

I've experienced quite a few memorable zone experiences in my lifetime. Most recently was during the M20 crossing where I felt like all systems were a 100% go and I just didn't want to stop. I was very aware of this state and it felt almost like a drug. It lasted longer then I have remembered it ever happening before, and I was stoked out of my mind. I was so happy I could barely contain myself. My crew on the boat could not believe the steady rhythm and strength that was exuding out of my every pore and muscle.

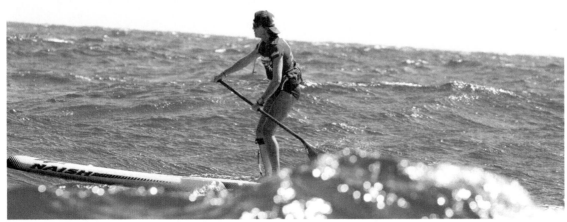

photo by Simone Reddingius

How to Increase Your Stand Up Paddling Performance

The funniest thing about that moment was that I didn't feel present. I mean I knew I was paddling hard and navigating tough conditions, but all of that didn't seem in focus. Everything felt totally in sync—my board, the ocean, and my body.

This has also happened to me while dirt biking and windsurfing when I landed some jumps or tricky climbs that I should not have made, and when I survived some waves in which I could have been totally annihilated. I don't remember how I did it, though. I just throttled hard or sheeted in, pumped the sail and flew.

HOW TO GET IN THE ZONE

If it has happened to you more than you can count on one hand during your athletic lifetime, consider yourself to be a person who is highly tuned into the state of your health, goals, focus, and performance. You also thrive in high levels of stress and excitement. It takes a trained mind to recognize this mental shift.

Annabel Anderson again kindly gave me her take on the subject as I posed a few questions for her talk about the zone.

For you, what does it feel like to be "in the zone"? Are you aware of your senses, your surroundings? Does it happen every time you compete? How do you define the "zone" or that sweet spot when all the stars line up during a heated moment?

Annabel writes:

"I have competed in many sports since I was a youngster. The older I get the more I realize that every sport/activity can require a different mental preparation to be able to perform at the best of your ability.

Personally, I am pretty in tune with how I feel mentally and emotionally and can sense the energy of my surroundings. By doing this I can adapt where I am on that particular day to where I know I need to be to perform.

This also means not treating every start line like it's the biggest event of the year. If you do that, you'll soon be burnt out and tired when you really need to 'turn on.'

You might as well plan on a race going wrong because there are so many factors you can't control (the actions of others, the conditions, course changes, weather etc.). If you can remain calm, you'll have a better chance to use your head and not get flustered—which will only cause unnecessary stress and for your heart rate to elevate.

The only way you'll get better at managing stress is to go and put yourself in stressful situations and develop an awareness of how you react during the heat of the moment. Identify what you do well and what you need to work on and then bring this into your day-to-day activities. Without practice you won't be able to use these skills when you need them."

Dr. Mihaly Csikszentmihalyi, world-renowned leading researcher and professor of positive psychology, originally from Croatia, has identified 6 factors or components that contribute and lend to the state of flow or being in the zone: [1]

1. An intense and focused concentration on the present moment.
2. A merging of action and awareness.
3. A loss of reflective self-consciousness.
4. A sense of personal control or agency over the situation or activity.
5. A distortion of temporal experience—one's subjective experience of time is altered.
6. An experience of the activity as intrinsically rewarding, also referred to as autotelic experience. (An autotelic experience is referring to a moment with purpose or meaning.)

He also states that these factors are usually present as you enter, during, or as you are ending your flow or zone moment, and they may not occur in any specific order. He notes that some of the greatest athletes of all times who continuously do well all exhibit these traits and states.

Reviewing the elements above I'm sure we all can probably relate to this in our own SUP training or race events. You can see how, when you enter the state of flow and you lose all sense of time, you forget about the pain in your shoulder, or how thirsty you may be. You may block out the noise or visuals from paddlers next to you because you are focusing on the task at hand—to win or do really, really well.

Next, in order for you, as a paddler, to get into this zone or flow, there are certain "conditions," as Dr. Csikszentmihalyi describes, that have to do more with level of intensity of the activity or goal at hand. For us it's increasing our SUP performance during a race or while training.

The activity must be one that is thrilling and exciting, not one that is static or boring, otherwise your mind will not engage at higher levels—it will be bored and complacent.

To set the stage for your zone and flow moment three things must be known: [2]

1. One must be involved in an activity with a clear set of goals and progress. This adds direction and structure to the task.

2. The task at hand must have clear and immediate feedback. This helps the person negotiate any changing demands and allows them to adjust their performance to maintain the flow state.

3. One must have a good balance between the *perceived* challenges of the task at hand and their own *perceived* skills. One must have confidence in one's ability to complete the task at hand.

In summary, the race or training session must be challenging and you must know how you want to finish. You will know immediately if you can pass a competitor or out-surf them so that you can adjust your stroke or paddle harder as the task calls (immediate feedback). Finally you must have in your mind the confidence that you are able to accept and conquer the challenge.

Here is a cool chart that illustrates the relationship between high and low-risk level of task challenge.

This graph illustrates one further aspect of being in the zone or flow: It is more likely to occur when the activity at hand is a higher-than-average challenge (above the center point) and the individual has above-average skills (to the right of the center point). [4] The center of this graph (where the sectors meet) represents one's average levels of challenge and skill across all activities an individual performs during their daily life. The further from the center an experience is, the greater the intensity of that state of being (whether it is flow or anxiety or boredom or relaxation). [5]

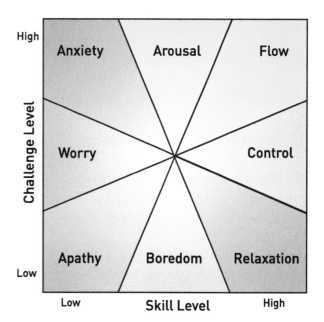

Mental state in terms of challenge level and skill level, according to Csikszentmihalyi's flow model.[1]

Keep in mind, we are all works in progress and all of ours skills are very different, individually, as are perceived challenges. This is just a reference tool to help you learn and grow your zone capacity.

Later in this chapter we will also touch upon how to manage anxiety, stress and other things so your zone experience will come more easily and more often.

THE OF TYPE OF PADDLER YOU'LL FIND IN THE ZONE

By now you may have guessed that it takes a certain kind of SUP athlete to transcend into this special performance state. You may already have in your mind some of the most disciplined top paddlers that probably seem like they've had lots of experience getting to and being in the zone.

Sure, some are blessed with lots of innate talent but I'd have to say that most have to work hard they just make it look easy. One thing they all have in common is their ability to focus.

With that notion I'd like to share a few example of those personality traits so you too can start thinking about your next or first visit in the zone.

Take Kody Kerbox, Naish team rider of many different disciplines. He does it all—long distance, surfing JAWS, channel crossings, sprint races; he's got experience in all SUP venues. Sure it helps to have good inherited lineage from that of his father Buzzy Kerbox, but to be able to perform at high levels time and time again, he's got this zone thing dialed—on his own.

I've had the pleasure of seeing Kody gracefully grow into the amazing athlete he is today—one with a finely tuned skill set. I've followed him for some time and now I get to help him achieve at even higher levels.

I know the signs for when he is in the zone. I see it watching him paddling (sometimes getting lapped by him) in the harbor doing laps with Bart DeZwart, Kai Lenny, and Connor Baxter, when I've had him on the beach, and while training in the studio. Sometimes when I've presented him with a challenging exercise or set I look at him and he has this look in his eyes as if he is there, but not *really* there. If only I could bottle that very moment and take a dose myself!

I often ask him, "Where did you just go?" He is not able to tell me, he just smiles big, because he knows he was there too, but his body did most of the work. That is simply amazing and very cool.

He is disciplined in all aspects of his training. He loves to learn about nutrition, makes sleep a priority, has confidence in his skill, but is still always wanting to learn more so that he can perform at higher levels. He is also patient and realizes that achieving high levels of success—in life and on the water—takes time.

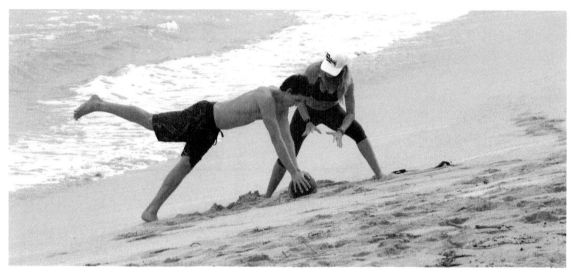

photo by Simone Reddingius

At the same time, he has a high level of confidence that he naturally exudes, but not in an all-knowing kind of way. He's had his wins and he's had his losses. Now, at a young age, he's well rounded in life thus far and that will serve him. No matter what the result is, he is always humble. Being humble and grateful are also great traits of champions.

Another client of mine, Bo Forster, a former ski racer and now paddler, also exhibits the same, intensely focused expressions. It is such a wild thing to observe. As she's in the middle of her set, I'll verbally cue her to push harder and it's like flipping a switch. She can immediately get herself in her zone with no problem. Then, as if I've snapped my fingers, she returns to "normal."

And lastly we look at another one of our favorites, Chris Parker of *SUPracer.com*. He paid a couple of visits to my Maui crib and I honestly think he thought a session with me would be a piece of cake. But Chris has got game and then some. He's always up for a challenge and, well, if you'd like to read more, here you go. Thank you Chris for being such a sport and such a support to the sport we love. Here's the article: *http://bit.ly/1PMIY1n*

The Boss Man, Chris, has a few seconds in the zone. Here's the photo:

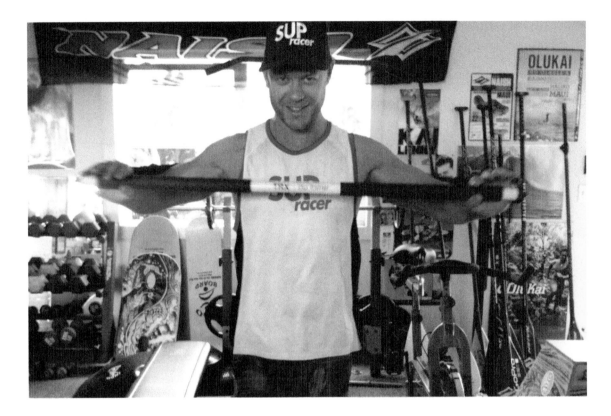

As a trainer, it is the ultimate joy to see an athlete perform like this time and time again. Even if I don't cue it up or verbally ask them to "go there," some do it on their own right at the precisely correct moment. Their eyes glaze over and their laser focus could penetrate a steel vault. Their performance is perfect, impeccable, and amazing!

THE COMMON CHARACTERISTICS OF ELITE ATHLETES THAT SPEND THE MOST TIME IN THE ZONE

I'd like to now cover some of the common profile or personality traits of the elite athletes that I've trained or observed in our SUP world. In general I think you'd agree that the some of the great SUP paddler athletes we know have many if not all of these shared qualities:

- Confidence: mental & physical
- Motivation/drive

- Defined paddling purpose
- Low anxiety
- High adaptation to adversity
- Passion

These are just a few; there are certainly more. As you look at these and think of yourself, do you see yourself having these traits too? Are there particular ones that you could do some work on? And if so, which ones? Which is the most dominant trait that you may portray?

Confidence: mental and physical

Having confidence reflects the beginning of the chapter—as we are now thinking like SUP athletes. The confidence you feel and display is a result of you anticipating success in your upcoming race. Your anticipated outcome is the greatest indicator of confidence. You are emotionally, physically and all knowing of your ability to crush it. That is the mental component of confidence.

The physical element of confidence is best formulated by Ross Tucker, Ph.D., Associate Professor of Exercise Physiology at the University of Cape Town, South Africa.

He explains that the brain's primary role during exercise is to regulate the body in such a way as to optimize performance while preventing self-harm through extremes in body temperature increase, oxygen deficit, muscle damage, muscle fuel depletion, and so forth.

When we are paddling in a long distance race the brain is prepared to enable you to paddle has hard and long as you can. It's a physiological strategy. Or simply put, your brain is pacing itself so it can help you do so without paddling yourself to complete depletion.

You might ask, "How does your brain know when you're about to paddle yourself into the proverbial wall, or as I often refer to hitting the end, as "red-lining," or "bonking?" (Refer to Chapter 6 for an explanation.)

Tucker states, "The brain is constantly receiving inputs and signals from every system in the body," and goes on to say, "and then interpreting these signals in the context of the exercise bout. It then alters the exercise intensity, by changing the degree of muscle activation to either slow the athlete down or allow him to speed up."

Dr. Tucker's preferred name for the physiological pacing mechanism is "anticipatory regulation" because it's based on an anticipated endpoint of exercise—the finish line. "The whole premise for pacing is that the brain is regulating exercise performance in order to protect the body from reaching a limit or a failure point or a potentially harmful level before the end of exercise," he says.

Motivation

This ties in with what I first touched upon earlier in this chapter. If you know your purpose or the internal "why" you have a certain goal, and you own it, you will be automatically motivated and driven from deep within your being. If, however, you are not clear and you are possibly motivated by external or extrinsic factors such as pleasing your boyfriend or a sponsor, for example, you may be less motivated.

Motivation comes naturally to the top performing paddlers because they are already committed and have defined their "why." They don't need motivation to train. It's innately in their internal programming.

Drive and motivation are almost one in the same. They can wax and wane but if your SUP training and expectations are in balance with each other it will be less work to maintain your motivation. You could be motivated to paddle better by several things:

1. Getting lapped or passed during practice or during a race.
2. Seeing someone new to the sport who is so excited that their enthusiasm just pours out of their body and reignites your fire too.
3. Coming off an injury and wanting to get back on the water.

As a trainer I have lots of skills to motivate people but I'm not successful unless we first define the "why" the person is training in the first place.

Defined paddling purpose

This is a biggie. All our lives we've been asked the questions, "So, what is your goal in life? What do you want to be when you grow up?" Now, we can go a little deeper because we're all adults (but we'll never grow up) and we've pondered this in our personal lives. Now we must uncover why we paddle. (And why you are reading this book, perhaps?) What is your SUP or paddling purpose?

Do you want to win as many races as possible? Will that fulfill you and pay the bills and meet the demands of your sponsors? Do you think by being the best paddler on the planet people will recognize you and make you feel worthy and validated as a person? Are you paddling for the enjoyment of SUP? Is your ultimate desire to share with your friends how awesome the sport is? Or are you paddling to get in better overall health? Is it a blend of a few things?

The answer to this question should include short- and long-term outcomes. You can re-assess and adjust as needed. Without this plan you will be lost and inefficient in your training.

You may have more than one defined purposes but whether you can list one or three, make them crystal clear and part of your mental mantra. Have that visual we talked about of you succeeding.

Low anxiety

From all of the research that I've explored, and especially with elite paddlers, I've come to the conclusion that there is somewhat of an inverse relationship between having high and low levels of anxiety.

Some theories postulate that low anxiety in the elite paddler helps one to be more resilient, manage a stressful situation better, be more emotionally stable, and, ultimately spend less energy getting worked up or worried about performance and outcome of the race.

On the other side, as we read in Dr. Csikszentmihalyi's findings, high levels of anxiety and arousal need to be present in an athlete's mental state in order for them to perform at high levels. Otherwise they will become bored at perform at low levels.

The takeaway here is that the way one deals with anxiety is an important characteristic of being an elite paddler. You'll learn, later in this chapter, how to manage your anxiety better.

High adaptation to adversity

Your ability to go with the flow during a stressful situation can cost you the race, or in more serious situations, can even cost you your life. I'm not trying to paint a dark picture here, but if you're faced with something totally out of the unknown and you panic, you can either have a great day or a really bad day.

Let's say, for example, you're venturing out for a serious downwind Maliko paddle and the swells are gigantic, the wind is ripping at 40mph, and all of a sudden your paddle snaps in two, or your rudder breaks and you have no way to steer and you don't know what to do or how to manage?

If you are quick to find solutions that means you are able to adapt to adversity or changing conditions, situations or both. You usually remain calm, assess, and go into action with the best possible plan, maybe adjusting along the way for a win or to make it to safety, or both. It's time to be the Buddha combined with a little MacGyver.

Elite paddlers seem to have this ability innately sewn into their fabric. I've seen many circumstances like the ones I mentioned above and have personally experienced several, too.

Years ago, during one training session on my usual 10 mile Maliko run, things on the ocean changed drastically fast. A system came in out of nowhere with huge, offshore winds and gusts to about 30 mph. I didn't handle things so well and I started hyperventilating and crying and thought I would never get back to shore. I thought I was going to get blown to Molokai. Luckily my dear friend Bill Hoffman talked me through and helped me keep my wits about me until we finally made it back. He taught me how to use my leg as a rudder. A couple of hours later I thought, "Well, if a shark bites it off halfway, at least I tried."

Now I'm much more experienced and try to help others when they're in rough situations.

You might also say that this type of paddler is more resilient and has the ability to be solution-oriented with the intense skill to focus only on the best way out. They do not give up until they find a way.

Passion

If all the above is true, the elite paddler will also have a deep passion for SUP and whatever is revealed along their path to their ultimate purpose. Passion brings enjoyment. You will see and feel this when you meet such a person; you may also feel the same way. It's so contagious and inspiring.

If you don't have this deep connection to the "what and why" that SUP brings you, then you might as well go count specks of sand at your nearest beach.

The actions you take and the words you speak reflect highly of your passion for stand up paddling. All of the hard training and the times that you fail help you learn and grow, adding to the passion that must fill you.

Just like in love, if the passion for SUP dies or becomes flat or stale, it's time to reignite that flame. Maybe try paddle surfing or teach a friend to paddle and get stoked off their stoke. You get the idea.

REMOVING THE BARRIERS AND OBSTACLES TO CLEAR THE PATH FOR SUP SUCCESS

You may have heard of the phrase "Lean in and let go." Does that seem like you? Or do you hold your paddle tightly, barely bend your knees, and are afraid of falling because you think you'd be deemed a failure if you did?

Are you a risk taker or are fear and anxiety holding you in paddle paralysis? I'm not saying go paddle off a waterfall, but I am saying, how about have a little more willingness to take more calculated risks so you get the chance to grow?

Do you hope or believe? Hope is wonderful but we must develop an expectation of success or victory. We must believe. Your belief fuels your willpower and the actions you take will lead you to success. Hope is not an action word and can actually keep you from achieving your goals.

Have you ever counted the number of positive and/or negative thoughts that cross your mind in a single day? Have you ever noticed that some people love to complain, find fault in other paddlers, gossip, and say hurtful things and you find yourself just wanting to sweep them away with your paddle?

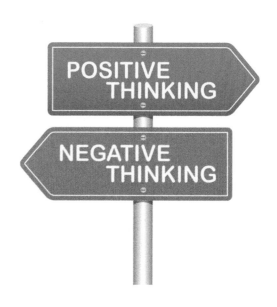

Are you conscientious of the words you select to express yourself or to others in a conversation? Are they positive? Or would you say there are more negative thoughts, worries, or shadows of self-doubt that, in turn, bring out your paddling and personal worst?

It's okay to acknowledge maybe a few times when you haven't felt the best about yourself. That's what makes us human. You could, at times, swear at yourself, calling yourself an idiot paddling fool. If you have done that, stop now! I'll have no more of that, please, as it's now time to learn new ways to think better of yourself of others. It's time to clear your own muddy waters to paddle positively with better mental SUP performance.

COMMON BARRIERS AND OBSTACLES THAT PREVENT US FROM SUP SUCCESS

It is my goal and desire to allow my clients, and you, the comfort and space to recognize certain real barriers that may be preventing you from reaching your SUPreme state of SUP performance.

Those of you who train with me or follow me on social media will, from time to time, see me post pictures of my white board with motivational thoughts. One that really fits well here, is this one:

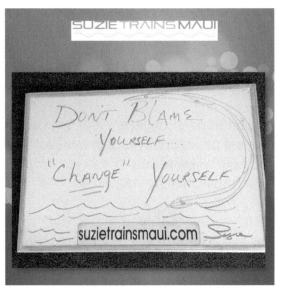

I really love this and I think it rings true for all of us. We have the power to make positive, long lasting changes in our thoughts and behaviors that will ultimately lead us to great lives and SUP performance.

It is simply amazing to me how many of us get in our own way. Though there are many points I could touch upon, I've selected my top five that I really think nail it. I hope you'll take the extra time here to do a little soul searching. These are not in any order but they are all related. You may identify will all of them or maybe just a few. It's all good, just keep an open portal.

- Negative thoughts, language, and people
- Low self esteem
- Fear
- Pre-race anxiety
- External distractions

Negative thoughts, language, and people

Do you know that the power of words can have a dramatic affect on the outcome of your everyday and paddling success? The words you speak or have in your thoughts shape how you act and react to life and how you paddle. Later in this chapter we'll have a little word play to help you reprogram so the days on and off the water are full of personal breakthroughs.

Also, to avoid paddling backwards or sideways on our journey, know that unhealthy, negative people also can have a great emotional influence on our lives. It's important to recognize them early and sometimes distance yourself. Paddle away from them now.

One of the things I've had to work on in my life is having thicker skin and letting things roll off my back, not taking on other people's stuff or taking things so personally.

As a trainer I'm also kind of a physiologist. Part of my job is to create a comfortable, confidential, safe environment for people to trust and express their needs and feelings.

It is then that we can work together to develop new languages and new words that transfer either good or bad. Language, meaning we often become programmed with phrases we hear from others. Words and expressions are passed along to the subconscious as early as 7 years old, and studies conclude these are the most formative years where we shape our entire life. We are like big sponges. Sometimes we inherit these languages unknowingly.

I'll give you my own personal example. I like to think most people have good intentions. Once in awhile a wolf in sheep's clothing comes along and unfortunately is not truthful or is simply on the take. I've always thought I had a very keen judge of character and I've always gone with my gut as it's proved to be right time and time again.

This person was a slick operator who said and presented in all the right ways and in the end took me for a financial and emotional ride, because I let it happen! My radar was on low and I was hopeful to make it a go. I was trying to look past what my gut was telling me. I thought, "Gee, here I'm handing you my world on a silver platter and this is what I get in return?"

My point here is this: I was a bitter pill for many months after and I had a ridiculous time of letting it go. I was hugely disappointed, disenchanted and felt wronged. The negative chatter that occupied my brain and personal space, ESPECIALLY when I was training on Maliko, crushed my spirit. I let it. I was not able to change gears, change the words, or change the language and negative thoughts I had of this person for many months after.

I allowed it to interfere with my life and my paddling performance. I felt like such a fool and idiot and then I was even more upset at myself for allowing this person to take so my space in my head.

Have you ever had this happen to you? How did you feel and how did you manage it? Are you the type of person that can just compartmentalize and not let it affect you?

I continue to this day to work on that. I have actually created clever tools and methods that I'll share with you so that you can re-route the negative words and thoughts and paddle off mentally stronger into the sunset or over the finish line.

Another example is that if a client says to me, "I'm have horrible balance problems and I'll never be able to paddle surf better. I just keep falling and I'm so sick of it. I'll never be able to do it," I say to them, "Well if you say so." If you tell yourself you are bad at something, guess what? You will be. If you tell yourself you have bad balance or can't catch waves, you will have bad balance and won't catch as many waves. It's that simple.

I then ask them to repeat after me out loud, "I am a good paddle surfer and I have good balance." They roll their eyes, but they take their turn and repeat it. Immediately at that moment, I'll cue them up for a challenging balance exercise. Okay Joe it's your turn again, "I'm a good paddle surfer and I have good balance."

By then we're laughing and I've just given him powerful words—words that he physically spoke out of his own mouth—that will hopefully reinforce a new, positive habit. The words and actions to reinforce those words have been stored in his paddle bank.

I could have told Joe that what he was saying was self-sabotage, but he already knew that. In no way would I acknowledge that or affirm his statements. I offered him new words and phrases for him to use as his mantra or new message to his sub conscious.

Trained SUP athletes work very hard at being their best, not just at stand up paddling, but in all aspects of their lives. I tell my clients and athletes to always surround yourself with people who are inspiring, supportive, positive and who help you shape your ideal thoughts and visuals of exactly how you wish to perform on the water and in life.

It's important to have healthy circles of people surrounding you with affirming, action-oriented words and thoughts. The top, top athletes regard their bodies as well as their minds as their sacred temples and they are very selective in how they train and how they live their life. Take note.

Low self esteem

Your actions, including your thoughts and how you speak and express your belief in yourself can directly affect how worthy you may or may not feel about yourself. Many times I interact with people that have been told that they are not worthy—whether in words and/or in actions—so throughout their entire lives that's how they roll. They've been trained to think they aren't worthy or able. This breaks my heart.

We may have all experienced this at some point in our lives or maybe you are feeling this a little bit now? Low self-esteem is really caused by warped messages that someone believes to be true. Usually it started in some form either growing up early in life, or later in life—maybe in the workplace—from getting bullied at school, or could be coming from someone in our lives right at this moment.

The result of this is that we become our worst critic, judging ourselves with scorn and negative feelings that ultimately take shape in every aspect of our lives, including on the water.

You might transfer the above feelings to how you see yourself amongst your paddling peers or in other social paddling circles. You want to be accepted but don't accept yourself enough to be worthy.

I encourage you to please reach out and continue to connect with the water if that feeds your soul and makes you feel good. Allow the wonderful community of SUP to embrace you, as I've seen happen around the world, and start to smile as big as you can. SUP does not judge; it is all about love. I mean that in the most sincere, caring way.

I also want to add that what you see on social media is not always "real." Don't compare yourself to all of the selfies you see of people having and "amazing" time. Sure, there are some cool places to paddle and many paddle things are rad but that's just the stuff that people *want* us to see. We don't see the real life, less glamorous side of most people because that won't get them "likes." I'm sure you get my point.

Fear

Right off the bat, I will say that fear can be a good thing, as we all need some form of internal barometer to help regulate known and unknown risks. Fear can also, however, put us in a state of paddling paralysis, which halts our forward progress.

I've often been fascinated by those big wave riders who drop into JAWS. They just point their board and go. What is it in their brain that just says go? What neurological and physiological connect or disconnect takes place at the wave or water's edge? The answer to that is for an entirely different chapter or book another day.

What the heck goes through their mind, if anything? To answer that question is Maui's own, **Loch Eggers**, one of the first legendary big wave surfers to paddle into JAWS. I asked him flat out, "Loch, were you ever afraid out there?" His answer was simple, "Hell yes! I was terrified!"

That gave me some comfort knowing that he was human but still maybe also a little bit crazy. I know Loch understands the difference between taking stupid risks and taking calculated risks. He studies the waves, the tides, the steepness, the winds; all logical approaches are channeled into the focus of riding the biggest waves while knowing the risks.

The true athletic component that makes Loch and other top paddlers stand out is their willingness to expose themselves to the outcome, be it good or bad. Bottom line, he knows when to the make the drop and when not to make the drop.

I think fear keeps us in check. It's a reminder you have to take into account the possible consequences of your actions, and not thinking something through before doing it can be disastrous. The flip side to fear, or another dimension is the idea that if you know you can do something and take the calculated risk, it still might turn out badly but you have thought it through and know you have a chance of making it. And you understand the risks.

As they say:

No Risk-No Reward

Now, the other type of fear is referred to as the fear of failure. This is a real fear that is not talked about enough. This could also tie in with a lack of confidence or low self-esteem. Failing, sadly, is not a word with a positive connotation, but slowly I see the pendulum swinging toward people embracing what failure can teach them.

As crushing as it can be sometimes not to place in the top 5, if we always win how will we learn?

Take for example the OluKai downwind race, 2104. I thought I had it in the bag and I was passing people left and right. I really thought I nailed at least 3rd in my division. I came off the water and ran that last miserable 100 yard beach dash and thought, "No problem," only to learn that I got 5th place. My heart sank and yes, I was honestly bummed, but I did not feel like a failure. Considering I have this ciguatera condition that is worse in the sun and when I exercise, I felt my "failure" was a success.

Remember Sidney, the client who, earlier in this chapter, shared with us the quote about doing the most damage to your body if your mind was in the right frame? Well, he told me that he hates to fall off his paddleboard in the waves. Come hell or high water he is not going down. He gets so tense and so intense that he refuses falling off his board in the surf.

I said to him "That's how you can get hurt. And, how the heck are you going to learn anything if you won't fall?" He sheepishly grinned, and said, "Yeah but I don't like failing." Oh boy did he get an earful from me.

I tell my paddling clients if you're not falling you are not learning. So my mind spins to another quote:

"If you're unwilling to fail, you are unwilling to learn."

The best paddlers get this and I hope this becomes a positive mantra in your life.

Pre-race anxiety

Earlier in this chapter I talked about one of the characteristics that an elite paddler would exhibit, and that is having lower anxiety thresholds. This is a true statement. This paddler shows up very aware of the playing field. He or she is well fueled and confident with a touch of stress to keep his or her centered in the body and on the board. Being a little nervous can be a good thing, as it's natural and allows you to check in and check yourself. It also ensures that you don't underestimate the other paddlers you may be racing against.

I have to tell you the honest truth. Right before the start of the Maui to Molokai channel race this year I was overwhelmed with a rush of anxiety and a case of the teeth chattering nerve jitters. I mean literally, my teeth were chattering.

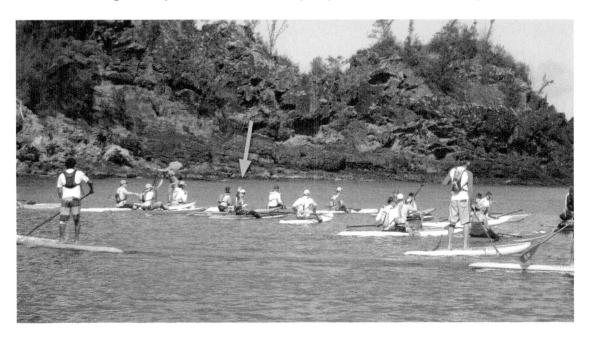

This was nothing new to me as it's happened a couple of times before I've headed out in big surf to paddle. But this time it was like one big shock convulsed through my body, and my teeth would not stop chattering.

I took deep breaths, looked up at the sky, shrugged my shoulders; whatever it took to "shake" it off. Wow. It was wild. Then I got the chills when we had 3 minutes on the clock until the horn. Soon I was up to my feet and going.

That feeling of being a bit on the edge, when it's hard to eat and maybe hard to sleep are all common characteristics of pre-race anxiety. One mistake I've seen some pros make is to go in too cocky and too assured of themselves only to find out that there were some pretty high-performing paddlers in the race that just blew them out of the water and off the podium.

What you don't want to have happen is to allow pre-race anxiety cause you to buckle at the knees or pass out before the race. I've seen people throw up in the bushes because they've worked themselves into a frothy frenzy and blew their cookies— literally—ruining their mental state right before the race.

Worrying yourself to oblivion does you no good, but having just the right amount of a little stress keeps your head on your body and in the game. I have tips in the next section on how to manage it so it works for you and not against you.

External distractions

We've been talking about internal distractions as possible barriers or obstacles that may prevent you from being your best, but what about the things outside of your mind?

We can't escape them; they are all around us. Cell phones, lack of time, lack of training, people, social media notifications, jobs, our real lives, and then there's static. I'll explain in a moment.

Identifying distractions and finding ways to divert them is a must. We all wish we could paddle full time for our real lives and some of you do! However most of us have other lives and other obligations that pull us away from precious paddling time. What else is there, right?

I tell my clients if you are a priority and your higher purpose has been identified then it's simple to start restructuring your life and quieting the external distractions so that you can hold your course. You are in control of most things you do in life, with the exception of severe weather, family emergencies, and static.

I refer to static as literally being external noise, television, or your computer. It would be nice if we could turn off people sometimes and have them talk to the hand. Kidding all aside, you have the power to quiet most of this—if you make the choice to do so.

TIPS AND TOOLS FOR STRENGTHENING YOUR MENTAL GAME FOR SUP

We've sure covered a lot here in this chapter and I hope that you are feeling mentally stronger and more knowledgeable by each sentence. Now it's time for the brainwork so that you can train smart and train right.

Before we get to the tips part, I really want to cover the definition of what it means to have **mental toughness** and **discipline** and being smart about it.

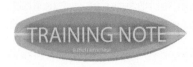

Training smart and having mental toughness is:

Learning to accept the burn but know the difference between scalding hot and burnt toast.

Some paddlers seem to have one or the other and some have both. Sometimes it is naturally hardwired while sometimes people really need to apply themselves with good practices. Mental toughness and discipline work together stroke by stroke. One needs the other to help you glide toward your own personal state of SUPreme paddling performance.

Mental discipline and training your brain for excellence has nothing to do with willpower and everything to do with believing you can achieve your goal. It has to do with the desire and knowing what the "why" is as you focus on your goal. You also have to have the belief that you can achieve your goal, adjusting your attitude along the way when the winds or waves don't set up the way you want.

Discipline is the time and sacrifices you are willing to make to put the time in every day and to move you to the end result. Are you wiling to get up every day at 5AM and show up, paddle, and train? Do you know how to balance your life so you can make the important time to do so? Do you have a list of excuses or "obstacles" that prevent you from being disciplined?

Once you develop these character attributes, next you need to have that staying power to stick to the program. Enthusiasm and the thrill of starting something new can wear thin, and the thrill is gone. Hold your course, be patient and stick to your plan that leads you to your higher purpose in paddling. Having a training partner is a great way to hold you accountable. That's another reason people hire me. You can bet I will hold you accountable and help you stay on course.

Determination is also a must, so that you do not to get derailed and follow through for the long haul, not just the short-term rewards.

Your discipline will soon become habit. Just as you have a deep connection to SUP and the water, you must also have a deep connection and an awareness of your daily purpose to get you to the "why." That is the definition of discipline.

I can't wait to see your success.

TIPS AND SUGGESTED PRACTICES TO HELP YOU GLIDE FORWARD

Managing pre-race anxiety

Don't let pre-race anxiety get the best of you so that you worry yourself right out of the race. Instead it's best to embrace it and stare at it in the face because, as we've learned, you need a little anxiety to keep you on your toes.

Examples of pre-race anxiety range from stomach jitters to shaking, shallow breathing, and feelings of being overwhelmed, declining confidence, and impaired judgment.

So how can you bring it down it notch and reduce some of the nervous jitters and butterflies?

Prepare
A few things you can do are quite simple, including, a few days before the race, preparing a list of things you'll need for race day. Get everything laid out and ready. That would also   include notes on your strategy and game plan.

Breathe
Next, learn how to control your breathing with deep breath exercises, preferably done in a quiet and calm area. Even if you're in your car at least that space is yours and quiet. The idea is to get yourself in a comfortable position, close your eyes, then nose-breathe in and out for a count of four on the inhale, and an equal count of four on the exhale. You can also get a meditation app on your smartphone.

Develop a routine
Having a pre-race ritual or routine is a great way to calm the nerves for some. Think about race day as just another day of training. You do this everyday and this is simply one of those days. You prepare your breakfast, go over your check-list, maybe sit for a while and quietly visualize the day ahead, and do some light stretching.

Stretch

Simple and gentle stretching can help calm your mind and relax your nervous system. Focus on each muscle group one at a time as you lengthen it. I'd suggest doing this an hour or two before your event. This could also be a part of your routine.

Positive self-talk

Letting any negative thoughts creep in can cause you to spiral down quickly and break down your confidence. Go ahead and tell yourself, "I'm a paddling machine." "You can do this." "This is going to be a great day." "It's all about having fun."

Expect the unexpected and learn how to cope

Not everything will go as planned so you need to have a head plan to get you through. Being resilient to adversity, chaos, and high levels of stress goes hand in hand with managing anxiety. But what is your plan B?

For example, lets say you bounce off or jam another competitor's board during a buoy turn and, all of sudden, you look down, and there's a gaping hole in your board. Sure, you'll think "Oh %@&!."

Don't let it paralyze you. Forge ahead and do your best. You'd be surprised how this could quite possibly act in your favor. You could be more determined than ever to win. Or, you could sit on your board for a few minutes, slouch over and cry. It's up to you.

Here's a quick story I'll share about what happened during my channel crossing from Maui to Molokai this year as for about 9 miles out of the 27 I had terrible stomach cramping. I didn't eat enough and had a hard time forcing myself. Then the wind stopped and I was paddling in a lake.

I thought to myself, "What?? Are you kidding me? You are the trainer. You are not supposed to cramp. You are not supposed to mentally crack. You are not supposed to have a meltdown." But I did.

The clock was ticking and I lost time. I lost my head for about a mile. I had to dig into the deepest part of my soul and pull my big girl pants up and shake the demons. It was the hardest thing I've ever had to do in a racing situation. Even in dirt biking, I've survived getting run over, losing a front tire off the bike, and crashing; I just got up, shook off the dirt, started the bike, if possible, and went on. This was, for some reason, extra difficult.

Even the best get injured or sick. Some of you are on the road so much—flying around with millions of germs ready to pounce. It's easy to get run down when you're exhausted from going back and forth between different time zones. How do you deal with that?

If you do get really sick, do you take the rest you need and emotionally accept it so you can be your best for the next race, or do you put on your stubborn hat and perform halfway?

I hear, time and time again, how some of you get your boards damaged, stolen or lost en route to an important race. You're tired and stressed and all of sudden you have no board. Your friends and sponsor are trying to find you a "like" board and you may end up on a board that just sucks. What do you do? Bail or go through with it? Those are tough calls sometimes.

You must expect a few small—hopefully not too many big—things to come across the radar that could interrupt your training or put you out of a race.

I used to work in the IRONMAN triage tent as a volunteer on the Big Island and also trained with the medical team the week before. We would be prepared for about anything to come our way during the race. But how well prepared were the athletes?

I'd meet the athletes and see them during that week before and then, sadly, I'd see a few in our tent right at the early stages of the race. Wow, let me tell, you the spirits in these athletes were crushed. Some were able to finish the race after we patched them up, while others would just about have a mental breakdown and not make it back to the bike or run, even though they were physically able.

Whether you have a mental and physical plan for the unexpected, or don't, and how resilient you are to preventing small or large unexpected challenges from becoming barriers is the difference between being a sub-elite paddler to a full-on elite paddler.

HOW TO PREPARE FOR THE UNEXPECTED

Control what you can

Go over your board, paddles, and leashes; everything you need for your race. Prepare your pre-race snack and fluids, and go over your checklist. Make sure you know where you're going, what time the pre-race meeting is, where to go for registration, and so forth.

Have an equipment backup plan. Not everyone has the luxury of having two boards available but you can maybe get two decent paddles in your quiver. You'd be surprised at what happens in the parking lot at races. I've seen paddles and boards run over and, worse, boards flying off cars before the event.

I highly suggest that you do not change anything in your routine, food, or gear the day before or the day of the race. This is where Murphy's Law will bite you hard.

Prepare your mind

Part of being an elite paddler is knowing how to manage your mind should something go wrong, whether equipment failure, harsh conditions, or your body conking out sooner than you expected.

You should know enough about your nutrition by now to be well prepared to avoid that. But even if you lose a fin or break your paddle, you still may have choices. Assess and decide: Do you finish? Can you finish?

Shift your thinking to "I can do this," rather than "Can I do this?" You may not be able to finish in the top five, but how awesome would it be to even finish the bloody race without a fin? You can't change an event, but you can control how you react to any unexpected surprises.

Stay as healthy as possible

There have been times that I've gotten myself so worked up for an event I could almost feel my body getting sick. Then I'd get more stressed and worried. You could wake up on race day with the flu, knowing you could do your best and risk getting even sicker before future races. Do you make peace with it and sit this one out?

I tell my clients, friends, and family, "If you are sick do not come near me." Avoid going to parties or large gatherings where germs are lingering and spread as half-sick people come up to you, kissing you on the cheek, or, through a hug, pass along their bug. This sounds very anti-social but you are guaranteed to get something. I put out an email to my clients a month before race day that says "Do not bring me unwanted gifts."

Take care of your body and guard it with lots of sleep, no alcohol, and minimal internal and external stress. This will help come race day.

Supportive and positive paddling posse

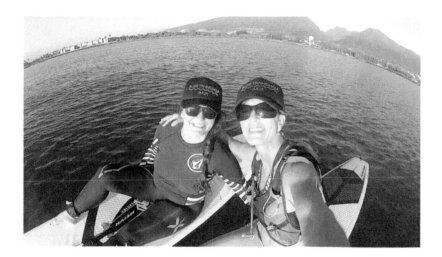

Stand up paddling brings forth such a welcoming vibe and is hugely supportive anyway; that's what attracts most of us in the first place. We talked about this earlier in the chapter—that sometimes we have to change our circles of friends for healthier, more supportive ones. Round up paddling buddies to train and play with. Finding someone who will hold you accountable can do wonders for your training goals. You will likely have no problem finding someone; just ask around and don't be shy.

Having a healthy positive paddling tribe is incredible and makes a huge difference in helping you stay motivated, inspired, and feeling good in your mind and body. That's one of the draws of SUP—the supportive types of people the sport naturally tends to attract.

Surrounding yourself with like-minded paddling peeps will also help you facilitate success. The smart SUP athlete understands his or her strengths and weakness and seeks help from specialists to help him or her work on certain things. Also, the sharpest SUP athletes don't pretend to have all the answers. They are constantly looking for new ways to sharpen their skill set or develop new ones.

Positive affirmations & action word play

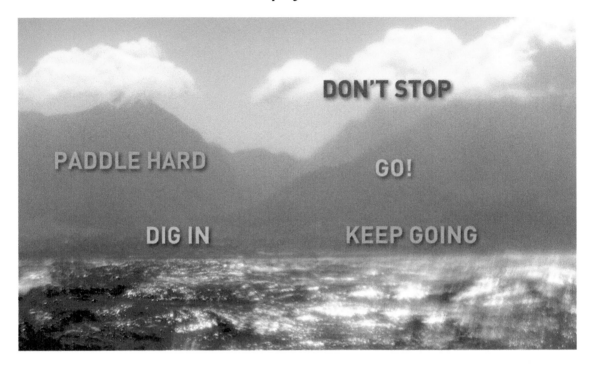

Earlier in this chapter I shared with you the fact that negative thoughts and words can create huge barriers in life that could hinder your success as a top performing stand up paddler.

The words you choose to express yourself will lead to positive feelings and actions. They must be turbo-charged and positive, propelling you towards your purpose or your "why." They will help you keep your path clear for SUP success.

It doesn't have to be just words. Your positive cues could also be images that make you smile and get you fired up! For example it could be a picture of you crossing the finish line at a very difficult SUP race. This is a great reminder that gets stored your subconscious. It could literally be just a big yellow happy face.

I suggest you create a subliminal word bank of your own and select your top three that really fire you up and keep you focused. Say them out loud, and place them in front of you on a 3x5 card to look at while you are training or while you are sitting a stoplight in your car. Or, better yet, make an entire deck of 3x5 cards that include visuals and words that get ingrained in your brain. The cognitive part of your brain will recall them when you need them.

I also highly suggest saying the words and phrases out loud to yourself. This is so powerful—it's really amazing. As you speak the words, stand up nice and tall with your shoulders back and head up. Say them over and over again.

First, here is a list of athlete action words that are directly related to what we do—paddling at our best:

Go

Paddle hard

Dig in

Keep going

Don't stop

These are just a few that might help. Now write down a few of your own.

We've all been there when maybe a few negative thoughts started to creep in like, "I can't paddle any longer." "Oh my God, I'm starting to bonk." "I can't go on." "Oh no she's passing me I'll never win." "I'm falling apart I can't paddle any faster."

How about these phrases instead:

"You can do this."

"You've got this"

"Suzie, head down and go."

"Breathe, go steady, breathe, breathe, breathe."

"Nice and easy keep going."

"That's right, strong stroke, steady stroke."

"It's okay, just keep breathing."

"I am a fierce competitor"

Whatever your phrase is, make it simple and clear. This is the mind endurance that will help you across the finish line.

Best practices to eliminate negative thoughts

Earlier I shared with you how this person whom I thought I trusted and had good intentions had turned out to simply play me and take my money? Well, remember how I said that I allowed this person to occupy my thoughts and energy for much too long so that it interfered not only with my SUP training, but also affected me deeply in my daily life?

Since then I've developed visual and physical cues that I'll share with you that I also share with my clients when I see that they are stuck on a certain task or goal. Or, if they are going through a personal crisis that is affecting their performance in the studio or on the water, I give them various cues to help them make a sharp and hard mind shift.

It's amazing how we hold onto the thoughts that hurt us. Some people can just simply put them in a drawer or compartmentalize an issue and move on. Not me, no sir. The harder I try the worse it gets.

So, when I find myself upset or distraught about something and I can't shake it here's my first course of action.

1. I will take this person or event and shrink him or her in my mind's eye. I make the person so small that he or she finally disappears. If it doesn't disappear I go to step two.

2. I visually imagine an old fashioned record player and, because I don't like that song, or our case this negative thought, I turn the dang record over. Next song.

3. If that fails, I take my hand out and put it in front of my body and make the motion as if I'm going to stop traffic in Paia and say the words out loud and very firmly, "Stop. Stop this thought right now." Then I pause and look at my hand another 5-10 seconds. It's amazing what that does. It really helps. Give it a try.

Suggestive thinking/self or professional hypnosis

For years people have thought hypnosis of any kind to be scary and only for the really weak. Not true. I am a huge fan of getting help to alter thoughts and change the dialogue in my brain that may not serve me.

Suggestive thinking is now kind of the new word for hypnosis and, if done correctly on your own or with the guided help of a professional, it can prove to be amazingly beneficial. You could almost describe it as to what could happen as you go into a meditative state.

The great thing about suggestive thinking is that you can do it just about anywhere anytime. It helps induce a relaxed state so you reprogram the subconscious with positive, affirming thoughts and words. Your subconscious is powerful and accounts for more than 80% of all of your actions.

There are many helpful techniques you can discover online or with the help of a professional. There are also smartphone apps that can guide you safely to a state of extreme relaxation so you can begin your flow of positive affirmations or suggestive thinking.

Suggestive thinking can be effectively used to

- Build your paddling confidence
- Reinforce newly learned paddling techniques
- Reduce pre-race anxiety
- Keep you motivated to train and push yourself
- Change a bad training or paddling habit
- Improve your self-esteem
- Help you manage pain

My own personal experience of getting hypnotized was generally good. I highly suggest you pre-interview someone or get a referral from a reliable source so that you can make sure their methods and approach are right for you.

I did have some success and learned some great cuing tools to help me manage intense pain. It was an interesting experience because at first I was skeptical, but I was desperate for relief. I learned a great deal about myself, and how I relate and cope with pain. So, personally, I got a lot out of it.

My closing thoughts for this chapter are that having amazing paddling skills and training hard are both important, but to achieve the SUPreme state of paddling performance, it is the mind that must win first.

References:

[1] Nakamura, J.; Csikszentmihalyi, M. (20 December 2001). "Flow Theory and Research." In C. R. Snyder Erik Wright, and Shane J. Lopez. *Handbook of Positive Psychology*. Oxford University Press. pp. 195–206. ISBN 978-0-19-803094-2. Retrieved 20 November 2013.

[2] Csikszentmihalyi, M.; Abuhamdeh, S. & Nakamura, J. (2005), "Flow," in Elliot, A., *Handbook of Competence and Motivation*, New York: The Guilford Press, pp. 598–698

[3} Csikszentmihalyi, M.; Abuhamdeh, S. & Nakamura, J. (2005), "Flow," in Elliot, A., *Handbook of Competence and Motivation*, New York: The Guilford Press, pp. 598–698

[4] Csikszentmihalyi, M. (1988), "The flow experience and its significance for human psychology," in Csikszentmihalyi, M., *Optimal experience: psychological studies of flow in consciousness*, Cambridge, UK: Cambridge University Press, pp. 15–35, ISBN 978-0-521-43809-4

[5] Snyder, C.R. & Lopez, S.J. (2007), Positive psychology: *The scientific and practical explorations of human strengths*, London, UK: Sage Publications

CHAPTER 8
Fueling and Nutrition Tips for SUP Performance Success

- Eating for SUP performance basics.
- Knowing your body's nutrient fuel consumption needs as a SUP athlete.
- The importance of hydration in training & competition.
- How and what to eat for proper SUP training and competition.
- Factors affecting a paddler's nutrition needs.
- My spin on SUPplements.
- Examples of real food for winning SUP fueling.
- Pre race fueling tips & competition wrap up.

Nutrition doesn't have to be difficult. Think of eating to fuel the engine that helps you over the finish line—maybe even onto the podium. Pull your board to the beach and take some notes!

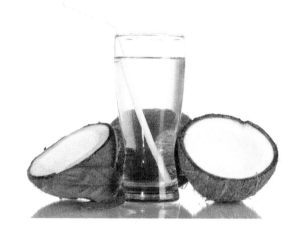

As a trainer and paddler I'm constantly hearing from people who are still seeking the magic bullet or "the one thing that works" so they don't have to think, plan, do, or know a whole lot about selecting the right food to help them paddle stronger and longer. They just want me to give them the short answer and they want it to be one that they like.

Granted, you don't have to be a chemist or scientist to know what's good and bad food, but maybe you just need some clarity and guidance to **KNSS** or **keep nutrition simple SUP** paddler. Right?

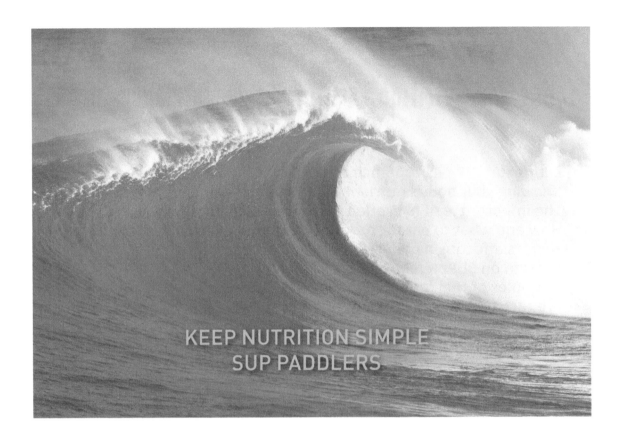
KEEP NUTRITION SIMPLE
SUP PADDLERS

THE WHY

Along with having the right SUP gear, having the proper fuel in your body is essential to improving performance and mastering the mental zone you need for success. Without it your stand up paddle performance will suffer.

Start by paying attention to your body's needs under all weather and water conditions and for all types of paddling. You can then fine-tune this aspect of your preparation so that you can feed yourself with energy-providing nutrients and food for endurance SUP performance. A short 3 mile race will require different nutrition than a 32 mile channel crossing.

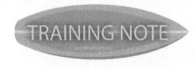

*I highly suggest that you keep a food performance journal identifying which foods work well for you, including amount of and which fluids you require and can tolerate during training and racing. This will complement your training journal. Don't forget to also record what you ingest after your training or performance. We'll get more into that later—the benefits of post-race eating for recovery. **Download SUP Performance Food Journal here:** http://bit.ly/1NOh7zg*

Also to *really* help yourself, track your weight changes and energy levels before and after paddling events, as well as intake of calories before, during, and after your performance. I've had some clients and friends take a scale with them in their car. They weigh in before and then after. (Keep in mind that levels of humidity can affect your water loss.)

It seems like A LOT of work, but in time you'll be able to fine tune everything and won't always need to write it all down. As you learn more about nutrition you'll hopefully learn to love healthy food that will help you give your best performance. Eating properly will become second nature to you.

Here is your FREE fueling performance journal download
http://bit.ly/1NOh7zg

You are, essentially, an individual science project, so there is no one formula, shake or diet that I can tell you to eat that will be the magic bullet. Your best plan may be a combination of several things you'll try and gather in your journal. I can't write the perfect menu for you, or suggest the exact right caloric to carb and protein conversion outcome for you, but I will offer guidelines and give helpful tips so you can figure out what works best for you.

This takes time, thoughtful planning, and a desire to learn and to respect your body as the one thing you just might have some control over. You don't have control over wave or wind conditions, but you do have control as to what you put in your mouth.

A LITTLE SCIENCE ON NUTRIENTS AS FUEL

Before we get into the number of grams and calories of this and that, I'd like to visit the three important types of nutrients that compose your fuel: **Carbohydrates, Protein** and **Fat**. Once we get a good feel for the basics of fueling, we'll start plugging them into some to formulas to help you determine your personal needs.

Carbohydrates

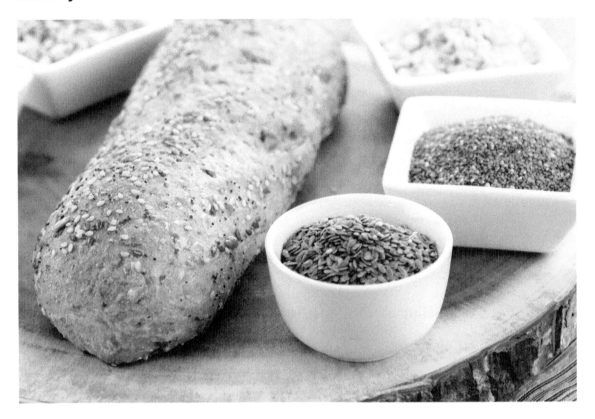

Out of the big three, carbs, protein, and fat, **carbohydrates** have a bad rep. However, because, out of the 55% of our daily totals of food we consume come from carbs, these are ultimately your best turbo power-boosting agent. For example

One gram of a carbohydrate supplies 4 calories.
Example: One Fig Newton has 60 calories per piece, 10 grams of carbs.
therefore
4 calories X 10 grams = 40 calories from Carbs
40/60 = 67% of your energy or fuel comes from Carbs

Unfortunately many people tend to reach for the bad carbs full of simple sugars, including table sugar (sucrose), syrup, sodas, high-fructose corn syrup, fruit juices, honey, and more. These types of carbs are also referred to as **simple carbs** or bad carbs.

Glucose (dextrose) is a common simple sugar found in fruits, some veggies, and honey. It's also the substance measured in blood. These simple sugars are low quality carbs and make up for empty calories that have little to no nutrient value.

People who constantly reach for the breads, sweets, and cookies are filling an empty hole with nothing but a whole lot of added weight, wasted time, and wasted opportunity. It is these carbs—that do little but pack on the pounds—that give carbs their bad name. The empty carbs are also truly disruptive in our bodies.

As a matter of fact, a new study that just came out (You can learn more about the evils of sugar by watching the great documentary on sugar just released called *Fed Up*.) stated that when rats were given the choice of sugar or cocaine, guess what they chose? SUGAR. It's the new brain addictive disease and it's wrecking havoc in millions of Americans. But not you, right?

Not all carbs are bad, though. There are good carbs that are an essential part of a balanced nutrition plan for athletic endeavors. Let's switch the science channel now and talk about the good fuel. These are the good carbs referred to as **complex carbs**, which you want to choose to launch yourself into complete SUP stardom. These foods are complex carbs: oatmeal, legumes, pasta, vegetables, quinoa, brown rice, beans, and more. (I will give you a great resource list a bit later)

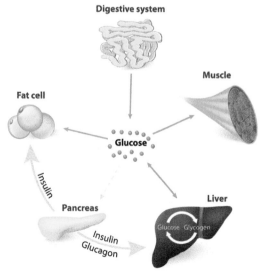

A really important carb found in your muscles and liver is called **glycogen** but is limited and can be depleted in about 3-4 hours of heavy paddling or training. The body breaks down most carbohydrates from the foods we eat and converts them to a type of sugar called **glucose**. Glucose is the main source of fuel for our cells. When the body doesn't need to use the glucose for energy, it stores it as glycogen in the liver and muscles.

During heavy paddling training sessions or endurance SUP races, such as channel crossings, you must increase your caloric intake—especially from complex carb foods—to maintain your glycogen stores and meet your energy needs. If you fail to do so while you're training a few things can happen:

- Chronic muscle tiredness or fatigue could set in.
- You could get a feeling of flatness or staleness.
- Unwanted weight loss could occur.
- Your sleep pattern could be Interrupted.

Now you know the importance of eating complex carbs. They are necessary to replenish the liver and muscle glycogen stores so that your heart, muscles, internal organs, and brain can keep their energy balanced and transfer it back to you when you need it most. This is a good time to reiterate the importance of starting your day with a good breakfast to maintain the energy balance and liver glycogen stores.

PROTEIN

Next, let's talk about the function of **protein**. Protein's role in a SUP athlete's nutrition program can be a bit misunderstood. Many paddlers still ask me if they should worry about eating too much protein for fear their muscles will get too big and slow them down. I'll touch more on that a bit later.

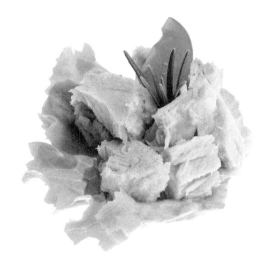

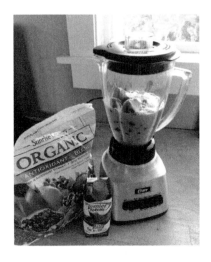

Proteins are large molecules that vary in size and consist of 20 amino acids (the building blocks of protein), which our bodies and the cells in our bodies need to function properly. Out of those 20, roughly 9 are called essential amino acids. The body cannot help make those so we have to get them through our food. Your body is kind of like a recycling machine, continually absorbing and using amino acids from proteins that you eat. As you digest food your body rebuilds proteins into the proper sequence needed for a specific task, which is pretty amazing.

Compared to carbohydrates, proteins are not a main source of energy but have a huge list of responsibilities:

- To help repair muscles after training or from injuries.
- Aid in muscle contraction.
- Act as a vehicle to carry minerals, fats and vitamins throughout the body.
- Direct energy production.

Below is an example of how much energy (calories) you can receive from protein:

One gram of a protein supplies 4 calories.
Example: Hard-boiled egg has 6 grams of protein
therefore
4 calories X 6 grams = 24 calories from proteins

Animal proteins are referred to as "complete proteins," as they are not missing any of the essential amino acids. Vegetable proteins (nuts, legumes, seeds and other veggies) are not complete proteins, but are still excellent nutrient sources and, as you learned earlier, they also bring some complex carbs to the table. That's a win-win! You can combine vegetable proteins in a meal to achieve a "complete protein."

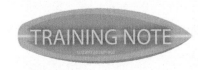
TRAINING NOTE

*The burning question remains: **Does more protein make you more buff?***

I'm not sure how this rumor got started but it's been going around for years and years that the more protein you eat the bigger your muscles become. I get lots of emails and inquiries about this as well and, while most people get the protein they need, and yes you as a SUP athlete may need more with intense demands placed on your body by training, the answer is false. Your muscles do not get bigger from eating more protein.

In the next section we'll go in-depth on how to determine how much protein you need to for higher levels of SUP performance. Please note that the extra scoop of protein or extra large helping of chicken or meat you eat could be converted to fat and stored as excess calories if you overdo it. AND if you get too much protein you can put unwanted stress on your liver and kidneys, which could then lead to dehydration.

FATS

Lastly I will mention the role of **fat**. As scary as that word may be to some of you it is the highest yielding nutrient for energy per calorie. Yes, if you consume too much of it, it will weigh you down, slow you down, and take a really long time to burn. It has its place in your nutritional plan, though. Fat is key for endurance paddling for long distance, while carbs help you perform better at higher intensities.

Fat is needed to help gain access to your carbs (glycogen) stores. Fat is our major form of stored energy and helps you paddle in extremely cold environments. It protects your organs, insulates your body, and provides structural support in your cells. Additionally, fat is necessary for the absorption of the fat-soluble vitamins A, D, E and K.

One gram of fat supplies 9 calories

The fat stores of the body are large in comparison with carbohydrate stores. In some forms of exercise (e.g., channel crossings, long distance races), carbohydrate depletion can cause fatigue. Depletion of these stores can occur within 1 to 2 hours of strenuous paddling. The total amount of energy stored as glycogen in the muscles and liver has been estimated to be approximately 2000 calories. Fat stores can contain more than 50 times the amount of energy contained in carbohydrate stores.

According to sports nutrition specialists Asker Jeukendrup, PhD, and Michael Gleeson PhD, ideally athletes would like to tap into their fat stores as much as possible and save the carbohydrate for later in a competition. (1) Enhancing fat metabolism, to spare carbohydrate stores to improve endurance performance is a common strategy. Learning how to manipulate one's own fat metabolic nutrition factors is a science in itself and has been proven useful for many.

Now that you have an idea of why fat is an important part of your nutritional plan here's how to identify the bad ones to stay away from and the good ones to use as fuel.

You've heard of the "bad" fats and the "good" fats? So in the order from bad to good:

- **Saturated:** "bad" very bad. Solid blob of fatty acids that raise your blood cholesterol which can lead to heart disease. Examples: animal fats in poultry, meats, and whole milk, and cheese are huge. There are a couple of exceptions here. Although most vegetable oils are unsaturated, some that aren't so bad but are still labeled at saturated fats include coconut oil and palm oil.

- **Trans fatty-acids:** You may have heard of unsaturated fats being processed as "hydrogenated" fats. These are everywhere and are often used as a food preservative or to change a texture of a food. This is when a liquid form of fat is turn into a semi-solid form of fat. Super gross and sadly don't, and are not required to, appear on food labels.

- **Monounsaturated & Polyunsaturated:** Both of these types of fats are usually in a liquid state at all times. Polyunsaturated fats are a bit better for you. Here are some examples of both:

    Monounsaturated: Most nuts, avocados, olive oil, canola oil
    Polyunsaturated: Fish oils, sunflower oil, safflower and soybean oil, corn oil, margarine, flaxseed

This gives you the basics so that you can be more aware of and examine your own food choices for fuel. You can see that to be an exceptionally fueled SUP athlete you need to know about nutrition.

KNOW YOUR BODY'S NUTRIENT FUEL CONSUMPTION NEEDS AS A SUP ATHLETE

It's obvious this food thing is very important and I really appreciate that you've stuck with me thus far. Determining the right amount of fuel takes planning, preparing, and figuring out what foods work the best as energy to fuel you. There are many variables that will have a significant impact on your performance and your fuel needs, including age, gender, genetics, and current level of fitness.

Fuel is also referred to as food, calories, nutrients, liquids, and, lastly, as "energy." How your body draws from your fuel stores is a science within itself.

How much fuel or energy (calories) will it take to fill your tank?

When you think of fuel for energy think food. To measure your energy needs think of a calorie. A calorie is a measure or unit of energy used to translate energy consumption through food and drinking to energy usage through physical activity.

It's not uncommon for some elite paddlers to consciously consume anywhere from 3500-5000 calories a day to keep up with their metabolic burn rate. Some even consume as many as 7000 + calories. To put it in perspective, the average male not seeking or needing to lose weight who is on a regular training program, may need about 2700 +/= calories a day, compared that of to a woman who fits the same profile would need about 2000-2200 per day.

One of the main concerns for serious paddling athletes is the importance of matching energy consumption with energy expenditure. Long distance paddles and sprint racing both require a large number of calories. Elite paddlers can potentially burn more than two to three times the number of calories as our new or less trained paddlers. If these calories are not replaced daily, over time the ability to perform during competitions will be compromised.

To find your ideal caloric or energy needs per day you need to first determine your **BMR**, or **basal metabolic rate**. (*http://bit.ly/1LVPa8l*) This is the rate in which your body burns calories at rest. Once you've got that information, next you'll need to figure out your activity multiplier, (see below) and select modifier of how much you work out, train and paddle. Then you will have a baseline of how many calories to approximately work with.

The original formula you may be most familiar with is the **Harris Benedict Formula. For ease of use you can quickly go to my website for this version of a BMR Calculator here**. *http://bit.ly/1NbvwWa*

Here is the formula, as an FYI:

MEN: BMR = 66 + [13.7 x weight (kg)] + [5 x height (cm)] - [6.76 x age (years)]

WOMEN: BMR = 655 + [9.6 x weight (kg)] + [1.8 x height (cm)] - [4.7 x age (years)]

Note: To convert pounds (lbs) to kilograms, kg:

pounds / 2.2 = kilograms
Example A women weighing 127 / 2.2 = 57.27 or 58 kg

A more up to date formula known as the **Mifflin –St. Jeor Formula** tends to overestimate one's needs, especially if you're overweight, but is a bit more with the times.

MEN: BMR = [9.99 x weight (kg)] + [6.25 x height (cm)] - [4.92 x age (years)] + 5

WOMEN: BMR = [9.99 x weight (kg)] + [6.25 x height (cm)] - [4.92 x age (years)] -161

Lastly, you can check out the **Katch-McArdle**, which can be good if you know your body fat percentage and are pretty lean.

BMR = 370 + (21.6 x LBM) Where LBM = [total weight (kg) x (100 - bodyfat %)]/100

Bottom line, if you know your body fat percentage, I suggest you select the Katch-McArdle formua. Also be realistic with regards to your daily activity modifier. Not everyone can be a 1.9 modifier! Keep in mind that you may train 1-2 hrs 3-4x a week but what about all the other hours in your day/week? You can always adjust, but it's best to be a bit conservative and real.

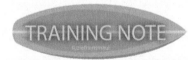

While no one formula or equation fits all please take the following factors into consideration when determining your caloric needs:

- *Current level of fitness*
- *Age and gender*
- *Health conditions, medications*
- *Total weight and lean mass versus fat percentage*
- *True activity levels, including daily life scenarios such as type of career and actual training time*
- *Diet and nutrient consumption*
- *Hormone factors*

Also please be sure to consult with your physician or qualified sports dietician should you have questions. It's important to note that a nutritionist is not a registered dietician. Anyone can call himself or herself a nutritionist.

Activity or Paddling Multiplyer	Your BMR Value:
Sedentary (little or no exercise)	x 1.2
Lightly active (light exercise/sports 1-3 days week)	x 1.375
Moderately active (moderate exercise/sports 3-5 days/week)	X 1.55
Very active (hard exercise/sports 6-7 days a week)	X 1.725
Extra active (very hard exercise/sports max 2x day training)	X 1.9

With all of this said, the *IDEAL* way for you to get your baseline caloric intake needs and to discover your needs as a paddling athlete is to keep a food performance journal for about 2-4 weeks. You can download my FREE food performance journal here. *http://bit.ly/1NOh7zg*

I know, from my own personal experience and success and that of others I train, writing down the information may seem a bit laborious, however those who did had a higher success rate in finding their true energy needs. It was also much easier to quickly have an "overview" because all of the info was right there for us to see. It's up to you whether you want to keep a notebook or use a phone app.

IF your weight is stable/ measurements are stable, you have likely found maintenance. You will track the following:

1. Date, day, time of day.
2. Energy level rated on scale of 1-10: 1 equals low, 10 means you're feeling great.
3. Food choice, including liquids.
4. Purpose of exercise--training, paddling, pleasure (be careful of mindless eating or grazing).
5. Portion: be as exact and honest as possible.
6. Caloric value: there are great smart phone apps to help you plug in caloric values.
7. Nutrient value in grams.
8. Duration of training, paddling time: hours and/or minutes.
9. Weight at end of week.
10. Personal notes.

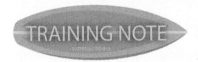

Here's a quick guide I give to my clients so they can easily get used to measuring their food without the fancy stuff:

Let your hand be your guide

One handfull: one ounce of nuts
Your palm: 3 ounces of meat
A fist: the size of a cup
A finger: one ounce

Take special note of how the food you ate sustained (kept you full) or not. Did you have enough or too much? This would also include all liquids too, including scoops of protein powder and their caloric values.

This does take time but I promise it will pay off in the long run. You'll be able to shape the best eating regime for your activity. You'll be able to fine-tune all your caloric and nutrient needs as you go. Having a history of your training and food intake in front of you is a great map to eating success and one you can continue building upon in the months and years to come.

Introducing new foods

Be careful as you begin to record and introduce *new* foods. Here is my own personal experience when I was experimenting with chia seeds.

One day I tried adding a small tablespoon of chia seeds in my water bottle to drink before I hit the harbor for some paddling laps. These seeds are amazing—high in protein, fiber, calcium, antioxidants, and omega-3s—but there *is* a right and a wrong way to eat them. You can put them in smoothies and yogurt or make chia pudding from seed that has had a chance to fully expand. Just be aware that these seeds also help food move quickly through your digestive track and are also touted to help you feel full longer, keeping you hydrated for endurance events.

If you are using them in your hydration pack or water bottle, allow them to expand first for a while *before* you drink and ingest them. You must let them soak before you ingest them because of how rapidly they can expand in your stomach.

Well, I forgot all of the above about waiting for the seed to expand, and, let me tell you, it was an awful experience into lap number one. Rounding the first buoy in the harbor I was doubled over with deep, painful intestinal cramping. There are no bathrooms there, except a scary porta potty, so I had to slowly paddle in, limp in with my board, load it up and quickly find a bathroom in town.

I also discovered that, in my attempts to add additional protein to my nutritional program, I cannot tolerate quinoa. As with the chia seed, I almost instantly get doubled over with cramping problems when I ingest it.

My point, I screwed up in my training, and since then I've been apprehensive to try chia seeds again. This is unusual, by the way, for a food reaction to be that quick and so violent. But you never know. What if I had done that at the beginning of a race? Yikes.

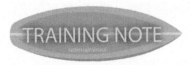 *I highly suggest you don't make any drastic changes before a big race or event. Do all the experimenting well in advance.*

Caloric intake in elite athletes

When I used to work with some of the IRONMAN athletes who would race in the Kona competition, a handful of these folks would come to Maui, train with me a bit, and in the same week as they are supposed to be recovering, would actually keep training for the Maui Xterra. Let me tell you—these guys and gals were eating machines.

During the entire few days they were here, they were consumed with finding their ideal food sources, eating, and hydrating as much as possible. They had dual purposes: They were trying to recover from one race, but at the same time they were rebuilding their carb stores.

I think out of the three I knew and worked with inevitably one, two, or all three would begin to get sick and run down. They all completed the races but not to their best abilities.

But one thing that's certain is that after all of the months of training and years of competing they knew their bodies. They had it down to an art—knowing how many calories they needed and how to time when they ate. That's something we'll talk more about in a bit.

As you begin to chart your food plan start to take note of what food combinations worked the best for you and what you might want to eliminate. You will also learn about your body's burn rate and fuel-replenishing needs, what you can and cannot tolerate, what to eat after training, etc.

Later in this chapter I will provide you with a chart that lists lots of healthy complex carb choices, proteins, and the good fats.

How many carbs does a paddling athlete need?

Once you have established a baseline for calorie needs we'll start with **carbohydrates**. Most health professional and sports nutritionists agree that the athlete needs to consume about 3.0-4.5 +/- grams of carbs per pound of body weight per day. To bring this into perspective, the non-athletes need only about 1.8-2.3 grams per pound of body weight.

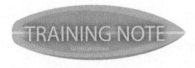

If you are exploring MET or metabolic efficiency training, carbs take on a whole new meaning. I will save that for another book. If you would like to learn more about this type training and how to maximize the use of your fat stores then this might be a topic for you to explore.

Your needs change based on duration of training or paddling. Using the chart below you can determine how heavily you're training or paddling then multiply the recommended grams of carbohydrate by your body weight to determine your daily carbohydrate requirement. During some long channel crossings you may be paddling over 5 to 6 hours so adjust accordingly:

Time Length of Training/Paddling	Grams of Carbohydrate per Pound per Day
1 hour per day	2.7 to 3.1 grams
2 hours per day	3.6 grams
3 hours per day	5 grams
4 or more hours	5.5 to 5.9 grams

For instance, let's say a 150 pound lean, elite paddler is training about 3 hours a day. We'll use 4.5 as the modifier.

150 pounds x 4.5 = 675 grams of carbs
Remember that 1 gram of carbs = 4 calories

Next convert 675 carb grams into carb calories by using the formula below:

675 x 4 = 2700 carb calories

So this paddler will need about 2700 calories in his day from carbohydrates to fuel him properly in addition to other calories coming from fats, proteins and liquids.

Carbohydrate loading: There are two schools of thought on this. If you're new to nutrition, carb loading is also known as "supercompensation" of carbs and glycogen before race day. The idea is to load up on huge amounts of glycogen, about 2-4 times more than usual in preparation into the muscle and liver for long endurance racing.

You'll notice that during an event they have the usual spaghetti feed the night before or that week. It's usually not a good idea to load up that much the night before but a little might help.

Just as you taper exercise before a race you can also taper your carb loading days. Check out this graph from the Navy SEAL Nutrition Guide below:

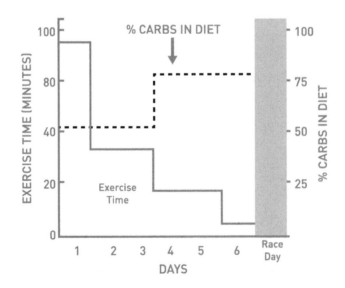

How much protein does a paddling athlete need?

Again, there are many theories and debates as to how much protein an endurance athlete needs daily to perform at their best. There's loads of varying data that can make you dizzy unless you are a scientist or have a degree in sports nutrition. It is agreed that men need about 10 more grams of protein than woman, per day, regardless of activity level. On average the general protein needs of a male are about 56g per day and a woman 46g per day.

Grams of Protein Per Pound of Body Weight	
Level of Paddling or Training	Protein Factor
Low to moderate activity	.5 grams
Endurance training	.5-.8 grams
Strength/full grind kine-intense	.6-.9 grams
Teenage paddlers	.6-.9 grams

So let's say you're a solid 175 pounds of power and your training and paddling is distance/endurance based most days. I'm going use the 0.8 protein factor of grams per pound of body weight per day.

Protein Needs = 0.8 x 175 = 140 grams per day

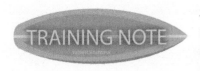

Some people have a tendency to go a little bit nuts on the extra protein intake, which often leads to unwanted extra calories and unwanted weight gain. I'd for sure keep track of this in your paddling food journal.

Next we'll touch upon your needs for healthy fat intake needs as a freak'n SUP amazing machine.

How much fat does a paddle athlete need?

If our overall fueling goal is to spare our protein nutrients to preserve muscles, consuming adequate calories from fat, along with carbohydrates, is important. A SUP athlete should consume 20 to 25% of caloric intake from fat.

To estimate how many grams of fat this would be, multiply daily caloric intake by .20 or by .25 and divide the resulting number by 9. (There are 9 calories in a gram of fat.)

For example, if you need 2,500 calories a day the fat intake should be **55** to **70 grams of fat daily**

(2,500 calories X .20 or .25 divided by 9.)

There's a lot of good information here and it may take a little bit to get yourself more comfortable with formatting some nice formulas for yourself. But, as I keep saying, having this understanding now will help you so much as a paddler go to the next level.

THE IMPORTANCE OF HYDRATION IN TRAINING & COMPETITION

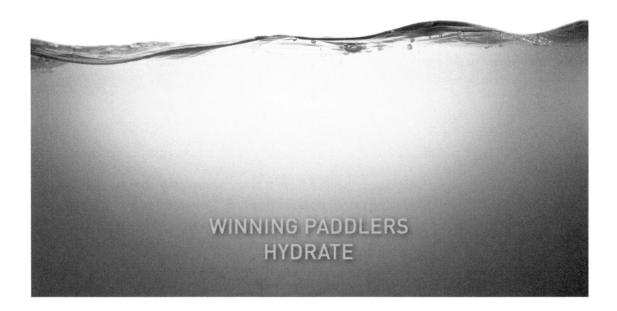

Most of us can probably recall one of the nasty hot, humid, or dry races or training days where we said, "shoulda, woulda, coulda," in regards to our liquid intake. Yup, me too. Hydrating properly is the one of simplest tools in our toolbox for our SUP performance nutrition needs, but often one that the easiest to screw up! I'm amazed at how many people I see who don't drink water when training or racing.

I think the hardest concept for people to get their head around is to drink even when you're not thirsty and then learn how to hydrate before a big training day or week or big event. There are so many cool hydration packs now that you barely know are there if you are fitted properly so there's no excuse not to take water with you while paddling.

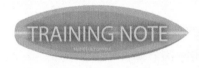

If you are thinking of completing a race lasting longer than an hour, or doing an endurance race such as a channel crossing, I highly recommend you carry an extra mouth nozzle in your hydration pack in case yours comes off at the wrong time. You could either lose all your fluids, and/or not be able suck out your fluids.

The other problem these days is a lot of our "sports drinks" contain a lot of crap, such as corn syrup, fructose, and other simple sugars; it's confusing to figure out what to select. Low quality energy drinks can possibly cause stomach and digestion stress. The sexy commercials we see tout claims that you'll be that refreshed and sexy too if you drink their drink; paddler beware!

Before I offer you some guidelines for what, how, and when to hydrate to achieve a SUPreme state of performance paddling, I think it's important for you to learn a little about how your body uses water, as well as what to be aware of—externally and internally—regarding hydration, and measures to take to ensure proper hydration.

If you're curious as to how much fluid you sweat or lose during an intense paddling training session, weigh yourself before and after. Hydrate as you normally would, go paddle, and then weigh yourself. Once you know how much water you lose through sweating, for every pound of weight you might lose, drink about 2 cups or 16 ounces to replenish that loss before paddling and after paddling.

You may have heard or learned that our bodies are mostly water, and that our total body weight is approximately 60% water. Here's another cool fact: Because lean body/muscle mass requires more water than fat, the leaner you are the more body water you have.

Water in your body provides the following important functions:

- Helps eliminate waste.
- Maintains blood circulation all throughout your body.
- Aids in the digestion and nutrient absorption.
- Maintains and regulates your body temperature.

Even if you lose a small percentage of fluids, even as little as 4 percent, from sweating, you can be left feeling disoriented, weak, unable to make important decisions, and you could lose your focus entirely. Becoming dehydrated can leave you feeling really, really sick.

Let's put this into perspective. Imagine a channel crossing or distance race if you begin to lose a certain percent of body weight, here's how you could feel:

	0	Feeling Pretty Good
% of Body Weight Loss	1	Feeling thirsty
	2	Increasing thirst; beginning to feel uncomfortable
	3	Dry mouth, urine output reduced; blood volume decreases
	4	Reduced physical performance; feeling sick, cramping
	5	Loss of concentration & focus, sleepiness, intense headache

Your performance can be greatly hindered if you are not in tune with your hydration needs. So next, let's review what type of conditions can increase your risks of dehydration:

- High altitude
- Travel
- Training or racing in extreme cold or hot conditions
- Training or racing over 30 minutes
- Drinking too much alcohol night before or performing with a hangover
- Lack of sleep

SUP performance hydrating goal: maintain normal balance of water

In order to stay ahead of the pack and on top of your SUP training it's important to keep your internal fluids (water) levels in check and not let them drop. When you become dehydrated your water output exceeds your input, creating a negative balance.

According to the Navy Seal Nutrition Guide a male needs to consume an average of .9 to 2.4 quarts of water a day. It's lost through breathing, sweating, in urine and in stools.

When you're having a light paddling or training day, most of your fluids will be lost through your urine. As you turn it up and the temperature goes up you'll sweat a lot more and could possibly lose about 1.8 quarts per hour.

Your goal will be to pay attention to keeping your body in water balance by taking in water from food, drinks such as orange juice, or, even, from smoothies. An example of foods high in water—some as much as 90%—include watermelon, cucumbers, and strawberries. Also, when your food breaks down a bit of water is released from the chemical process. In the end, staying hydrated by drinking good, old-fashioned water is best.

What to drink

There is a bit to know about proper hydration for SUP racing and training. I know some of you reading this really take this to heart and do a great job. Some of you may be learning new information and might toy with the notion, "more is better?" Stop right there. Did you know that some novice to intermediate endurance athletes have tendencies to *over* hydrate which can lead to severe physiological circumstances, including death? *Now I've got your attention!*

I've seen it all while volunteering for several years on the Big Island at the IRONMAN event in the triage tent. Wow, what a scene! Our cots were constantly full with disappointed athletes as our team worked hard to stabilize them quickly--back to a "normal" state.

Some of these athletes train their entire life for this event and blow up, usually from under hydrating, though on rare occasions you see an unusual case where an athlete has over hydrated; both leading to a condition called hyponatremia (low blood sodium). It's painful and can cause intense muscle cramping, severe bloating and uncomfortable urine deletion.

Let's discuss quality of drink selection. There is a term that many of you may have never heard before and that is **osmolality**, or particles per liter. The lower the number of particles in a solution (the lower the mOsm/L) per liter the better. The higher measurement (particularly if it's above 350) of mOsm/L the greater risk for stomach problems. As a SUP athlete you already know quality in equals quality out. Not all sports drinks or fluids we choose are high in *mOsm/L*.

As stated by James Wesley M.S. Forensic Chemist, Clinical Toxicologist, Rochester, NY for a paper titled Sports Hydration 07, "The kidneys control the retention and excretion of water and sodium in order to keep the body in a state of fluid balance, indicated by the overall combined levels of dissolved salts, sugar and other solids called the **osmolality. *A normal osmolality is 282-295 mOsm/kg***. When sweat causes **dehydration**, the plasma sodium and osmolality increases, causing the antidiuretic hormone vasopressin to be released, resulting in the kidneys excreting sodium and retaining water. This process continues until the high osmolality is reduced to normal. The athlete also gets very thirsty, because drinking water also lowers the plasma osmolality."

Normally, when an athlete (or anyone) drinks too much water or sports drink, little vasopressin is released and the kidneys retain salt and excrete water, producing large volumes of dilute urine. This response continues until the low osmolality increases and becomes normal again."

If you choose a sports drink that is high in osmolality, such as Gatorade, which ranges from 280-260 particles per liter, you can dilute it with equal parts water to avoid problems. Other examples of fluid replacement drinks that tend to also have super high levels of fructose, sucrose and corn syrup would be Coca Cola (600-715) and orange juice (690). Funny, I do know some endurance athletes love a nice cold Coke!

The reason I bring all this up about osmolality is to help you understand that our blood has a state of plasma composition osmolality, and according to Peak Performance specialists of Canada, this is a measure of the concentration of sodium, chloride, potassium, glucose and other ions (molecules with a positive or negative electric charge) in the blood. This osmolality is affected by changes in water content, increasing with dehydration and decreasing with over hydration. Normal plasma osmolality ranges from 275-300 mOsm/kg. This is similar to the osmolality of sport drinks.

The kidneys play a protective role in the hydration status of the body. Kidneys help to regulate plasma osmolality by reabsorbing water when we are dehydrated and increases filtration rate when we are overhydrated. Although the composition of sweat varies from person to person, it is always hypotonic (less concentrated) compared to body fluids, and therefore sweat loss increases plasma osmolality.

Now you know why that electrolyte concentration of sodium, chloride, potassium and glucose are so important to replace as we perform. What you choose to drink for your training—before, during, and after a SUP race or intense training session is important.

Drinking sports drinks is an easy way to replace water, carbohydrate, and sodium losses incurred during and after paddling or training. Replacing the large amounts of sodium lost in sweat may help you avoid hyponatremia. Peak Performance of Canada also suggests consuming glucose-electrolyte solutions, with a hypotonic osmolality compared to plasma, to help maximize the rate of water uptake.

They also conclude that the type of sugar in sport drinks may also have an effect on absorption. Research shows that glucose stimulates more net water and sodium absorption than does fructose. Maltodextrin, a glucose polymer often found in sport drinks, might be the most effectively absorbed. It is less sweet than glucose or fructose, and is often mixed with other sugars to increase palatability. Maltodextrin refers to a family of glucose polymers, is composed of between 3-19 molecules of glucose, and is commercially manufactured from potato, corn, or rice.

Now that you have all of this juicy hydration information, you can start researching more in-depth the quality of what you put in that fine paddling body of yours. I want to see you at the finish line, not on the sidelines, or, worse, in the medical tent.

My hydration picks

I've spent some time experimenting and trying to figure out my own hydration needs. For me it depends length of SUP race, expected conditions (humid or baking hot) and, most importantly, what my stomach can easily digest and tolerate.

Personally, I LOVE Amy and Brian's Coconut Juice, but it's the same thing as coconut water. Coconut water has nice levels of potassium, good carbs, and is low in sugar.

For races or hard training under 2 hours I may use a half scoop or full scoop of HEED by Hammer Products per liter of water. I'm really sensitive so I tend to use a lot less than is recommended. For races or channel crossings I will use Perpetuem, another Hammer Product, but adjust accordingly because my stomach can't tolerate the normal recommended amounts. I pre-mix one liter bottles so they are ready and on hand.

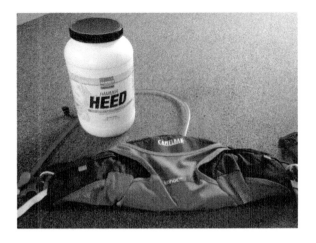

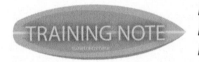 *If paddling in super hot conditions or if your race starts in the heat of the day, you can freeze your hydration bladder over night with your fluid mixture. Works well to keep your fluids nice and cool.*

I made the mistake once of letting my boyfriend Tommy, who was trying to help, pre-mix my hydration pack with too much of my electrolyte drink. Oh my gosh, did he overload me! It was a bad mistake because this particular downwind race had NO wind and a sticky icky lame swell. I felt like we were paddling backwards for ten miles with high levels of humidity. One small sip and I felt like I would puke. I had 9 miles of ten to go and I thought my head was going to pop off my body. BIG lesson learned. I had no fluid to drink and I think I saw a few unicorns dancing on the water as a result. LESSON: Manage my own fuel from here forward.

Here is a quick summary of some popular sports energy drinks and their value to you as a SUP athlete. Don't be fooled by some of the brands you see on the shelf. Some of these companies are owned by big brand soft drinks!

Beverages	The Good	Not So Good	Examples

Water	* Hydration
	* No calories
		* Low electrolyte and carbohydrate content
		* If bottled is environmentally unfriendly
			*Tap
			*Bottled
			  Evian
			  Dansi
			  Hawaiian
			  Figi

Coconut Water	**Hydration** *Full of vitamins & minerals Contains natural electrolytes * Good source of fiber * Per cup: 46 calories, 9+ g CHO, 0.5g fat * Tastes great		*Amy & Brian's *Vita Coco *Zico *Naked
Sports Drinks	* Hydrator * Electrolytes * Carbohydrate (sugar) for post- exercise recovery	* High in calories for inactive people * Can also be high in fructose	* Gatorade * Powerade * All Sport * Cytomax
Energy Drinks	* Central-nervous system stimulant * Ergogenic properties	* Most kinds contain caffeine * Not suitable for children *Less sustaining * High amounts of chemicals *Make you jittery	* Red Bull * Hype * Monster
Vitamin Water or "Enhanced Water"	* Hydration	* Mostly sugars, artificial colors, and flavors * Contains electrolytes but not sodium * Added Vitamins are not necessary- these vitamins are easily obtained through diet	* Glaceau vitamin water * Penta

Simple homemade electrolyte rehydration sports drinks

Your body's charging system relies on the positive effects of electrolytes to keep the body fueled and functioning. When the minerals in our bodies are out of balance things will break down very quickly, affecting the nervous system, how our muscles contract, and more.

I've done lots of research so that I could make my own hydration electrolyte drink. By having a few simple ingredients in the cupboard, including sea salt, baking soda, and sugar or a little high quality honey, you, too, can make the perfect liquid electrolyte drink.

Here are a couple of easy recipes:

1. Provided by the World Health Organization: This first recipe includes:

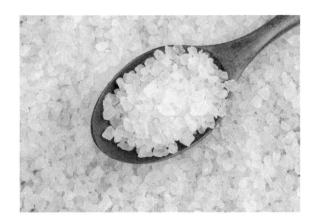

sodium chloride
trisodium citrate
potassium chloride
sugar/glucose
water

Ingredients:

½ tsp sea salt
¼ tsp baking soda
7 c of water
½ c fresh squeezed lemon juice
1 Tbsp of lime juice
¼ c of high quality organic honey

Note: *Baking soda contains sodium chloride, which is different than salt and our bodies need both.*

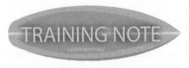

According to Livestrong(3), strenuous exercise leads to the buildup of lactic acid and the associated muscle pain and fatigue. The longer an athlete can delay lactic acid buildup, the better his performance, especially in situations that require endurance. That's exactly what drinking baking soda does for athletes. Baking soda has been found to be effective in boosting multiple sprint performances by neutralizing lactic acid buildup, thereby delaying muscle pain and fatigue.

---

2. Simple solution

The most basic hydration recipe combination is drinking water mixed with a 10-1 ratio of sugar to sea salt. Instead of sugar, you can use a natural sweetener, such as honey. Stir the drink until the salt and sugar are fully dissolved. Add a slice of lemon or lime to make it tastier.

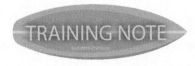

People often ask me if caffeine can cause dehydration? According to Katherine Zeratsky, R.D., L.D., contributing author at the Mayo Clinic, "Drinking caffeine-containing beverages as part of a normal lifestyle doesn't cause fluid loss in excess of the volume ingested. While caffeinated drinks may have a mild diuretic effect — meaning that they may cause the need to urinate — they don't appear to increase the risk of dehydration." Still, caffeinated drinks can cause headaches and insomnia in some people. Water is probably your best bet to stay hydrated.

How much to drink

Like everything in regards to fueling your body with food and fluids, not one formula will be right for everyone. Being as disciplined as possible when it comes to hydration can make such a difference for a successful SUP performance.

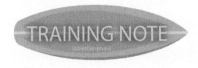

SUP Performance starts to decline when you lose 3 percent of your body weight in sweat. Beyond 3 percent your paddling performance can drop even more suddenly.

I often scratch my head when I see some paddlers just going for a training session that I know will be over an hour plus without water. Doing this is not macho at all and robs your body blind of precious minerals. If you can remember one thing it's this: drinking fluids before, during, and after a race or training session is super important.

Before we start taking ratios and how much and when, please review these quick tips to get you started:

- To get used to drinking water and/or more liquids, carry with you at all times a liter of water and drink, then refill. Get your bladder used to drinking maybe a little more then you may be used to if you're just getting into this nutrition thing. *Remember, even if you're not thirsty best to keep sipping at regular intervals in smaller quantities.*

- If you're paddling for less than an hour, you'll be fine drinking just water. Your body's own stores of carbohydrates and electrolytes are adequate to carry you for at least that long.

- Keep an eye on the color of your urine. The more clear the urine, the more hydrated you are. Note that certain supplements, vitamins or medications may have an effect on the color.

- To help reduce overheating wear appropriate clothing to help keep your engine inside cool. (Hat, light colored clothing, breathable fabrics)

- If you're doing a crossing with a relay partner, take advantage of your breaks by putting cold washcloth on nape of neck. It's awesome and can make a huge difference.

- As we've talked about over doing it, don't over hydrate. You've learned this can lead to serious and even fatal results. If you feel water sloshing around and feel super bloated stop. Risks are small for hyponatremia but don't risk it.

Suggested liquid intake guidelines

According to the Journal of Athletic Training, to help establish proper pre-hydration for athletic performance one should consume approximately:

500 to 600 mL (17 to 20 fl oz) of water or a sports drink 2 to 3 hours before exercise and 200 to 300 mL (7 to 10 fl oz) of water or a sports drink 10 to 20 minutes before exercise.

Fluid replacement should approximate sweat and urine losses and at least maintain hydration at less than 2 percent body weight reduction. This generally requires 200 to 300 mL (7 to 10 fl oz) every 10 to 20 minutes. (4)

To figure out your **normal daily needs** of fluids while not exercising or training:

Simply multiply your body weight in pounds by 0.5-0.6, which will give you the figure, in fluid ounces, that you should aim for daily. This is a bit more accurate than what we've heard for years—to drink 8 cups of water per day.

To **determine more precisely** how much you need during training:

Weigh in before 30-60 minutes and weigh in immediately after. I've seen people bring scales in the parking lot, no lie. Just keep your bathing suit or surf trunks on! If you lose up to a pound or more, you've lost fluids through sweat, so drink about 16 ounces to replenish. If you lose 2 pounds, then drink 32 ounces of fluids, and so forth.

If you lose a pound each time you train or paddle for 30 minutes replenish with 16 ounces of fluids.

Do this for at least 3-4 consistent training sessions and you'll be able to dial in your hydration needs.

When you are recording this data, make special note of the following:

- Outdoor conditions (temperature, humidity, etc.)
- Time of day
- Size or capacity of water bottle or bladder of hydration pack
- Time on water or training
- Level of exertion/intensity
- Average sweat rate from scale reading
- Paddling conditions: chop, wind in face, side swell, flat water
- Electrolyte consumption: what you used/portions
- Weight before/after

Recovery hydration

Recovering from an intense training session or a grueling SUP race is as important as preparing for one. Don't confuse recovery drinks with sports drinks. This is where many of us could probably do a bit better. This is SO important if you are on tour with races back to back or in consecutive day rounds. If you're only training or at it for about an hour or less, drinking water is fine.

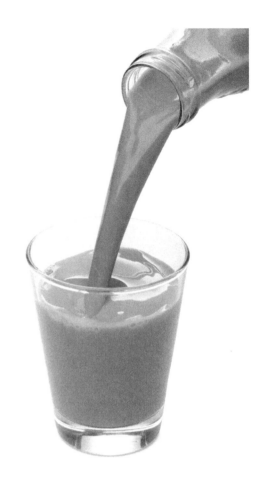

However, in order for you to get your body back to fluid balance as fast as possible, it's a good idea to think carbs and a little protein. The standard ratio of carbs to protein is 4:1, as together they bind well and allow your body to build back its muscle glycogen. The carbs will help steadily increase your energy so that you don't crash and gorge at your first meal and the protein will help fill you up and allow your muscles to begin repairing themselves.

Again, the more you practice, the more you will learn about what your body needs.

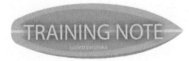

Just a note that ingesting too much protein can slow your body's process of replenishing glycogen stores.

Recovery Drinks	The Good	Not So Good	Examples
Water Usually fine alone if under 60 min in normal weather conditions	* Hydration * No calories	* Low electrolyte and carbohydrate content * If bottled is environmentally unfriendly	*Tap *Bottled Evian Dansi Hawaiian Figi
Chocolate Milk 8oz 1%	*3:1 ratio Carb:Protein *potassium 530mg *protein *32g DHA Omega-3 *sodium *fast absorbing	*possible allergy to dairy *not as easy to digest after intense exercise	*Horizon Organic Lowfat Chocolate Milk
Coconut Water	*high potassium	*Little sodium to help stabilize normal levels. *No protein	Amy & Brian's
Recoverite	*3:1 ratio Carb:Protein *Contains Maltodextrin, a glucose polymer, fast absorbing * good tasting *easy to digest	*lower in potassium	Hammer

HOW AND WHAT TO EAT FOR PROPER SUP TRAINING AND COMPETITION

Before, during, and after

Knowing the ins and outs of what to eat *before, during, and after* competition or training can be a bit confusing. Nutrition fads and trends go up and down like the size and widths of SUP surf boards. For example, some say pasta loading is old school and others still include as part of their pre-race food plan. I'd like to help make it as simple as possible. As I mentioned I am not a nutritionist nor will one suggestion fit all of you.

Before

I don't need to know what you ate 4 months before your event but let's keep it simple and say the week of and morning of race day. I'm assuming by now you've done your experimenting because it's part of your training. If you wait until race day you may be in big trouble.

ONE WEEK PRIOR: Besides calming nerves, tapering down your training, and all of the other details you need to manage for your big day, food should be THE priority. You need not eat less as your training decreases due to tapering. You can always use a little extra "calorie storage." Say no to alcohol, high sodium foods, sugar, and heavy foods high in fat. Focus on keeping a clean machine.

Carbohydrates
According to Nancy Clark, RD and author of the best-selling *Nancy Clark's Sports Nutrition Guidebook*, "If you plan to compete for longer than 90 minutes, you want to maximize the amount of glycogen stored in your muscles because poorly fueled muscles are associated with needless fatigue. The more glycogen, the more endurance (potentially)."(5) Her point: keep the carbs coming.

As you maintain your carb loading be careful not to overdo it with too much fruit or too many fibrous foods (to avoid diarrhea) and stay away from anything white such as white bread or rice that could clog you up. Speaking to the 'fat" of our topic, avoid butter on your roll, but maybe have two plain rolls. Swap out cheese on your pasta and stick to a light tomato sauce, and choose low-fat yogurt, not ice cream.

Protein
Although carbs are usually the primary focus, for SUP endurance races over 2-3 hours always add a small portion of protein to each meal to keep your body from eating its own muscles. This is referred to as lean muscle tissue catabolism or muscle cannibalization. This sounds gnarly and it is gnarly, as it can increase your ammonia levels, resulting in horrible performance effects. Some good protein choices include low-fat yogurt, turkey, chicken, lentils (easy to digest) and, potentially, some plant proteins including kale or tofu.

Fluids
Keep the fluids flowing and, of course avoid all booze, to prevent dehydration and other performance related issues. Drink as much as necessary to produce a steady flow of urine output on and off for about 2 hours. Make sure it's a pale yellow color. Watch out for too much caffeine as it can act as diuretic. No need to go too crazy on over hydrating. Remember what we talked about earlier and the disastrous affects of hyponatremia? (Too much water/fluids lowers natural levels of sodium and electrolyte levels.)

DAY BEFORE: People get all freaked out and over think this part and end up pigging out and feeling like crap all night and wake up sometimes with a high carb food hangover. Not good.

Think of this day as THE most important food day. Simply put, start with a light breakfast to include more carbs, such as a high quality multi-grain cereal with a sliced banana, and soy or low-fat milk, protein like a hardboiled egg and few ounces of turkey. You can swap the cereal for a couple of slices of high grain toast with almond butter.

Lunch should be the biggest meal so you can have time to store and digest. If you want to carb load, do it here instead of the night before. Don't over stuff yourself. I'm not going to tell you how many cups of pasta to eat, as you should have figured this out during your "training" sessions. When in doubt, less is more.

Remember to keep the pasta clean. Avoid high fat Alfredo sauces. Stick to marinara or light tomato sauce with no Parmesan cheese. You can have a little bit of olive oil so the noodles don't stick. If you want more flavor, add some chopped basil and/or oregano or thyme. You can add a small side salad with a small amount of chicken or hard-boiled egg. Sprinkle a few walnuts or sunflower seeds on top, a drizzle of balsamic vinegar and one of olive oil, finishing with a dash of pepper to taste.

For dinner, consider a small serving of brown rice or couscous with a small portion of lean meat such as fish or chicken. Maybe include a small bowl of low-fat yogurt topped with organic berries as a nice treat.

MORNING OF: Take a deep breath; it's go time. If you drink coffee, have a cup. We don't want you to suffer from a "caffeine headache." Let's say your race is at noon. Even if you are nervous you must eat. Plan the night before to have everything out on the counter and ready—food and gear. Leave yourself a note if there are things in the refrigerator that you're likely to forget.

Keep it light and filling to sustain you. I like to eat, 3-4 hours before if possible, one and a half cups of oatmeal with a dash of brown sugar and a banana. I also drink one coconut water to increase my potassium levels. In addition, I may drink a couple of glasses of water.

If I start to get a hunger pang before the race, I'm going to reach for what works best for me and that's one packet of Pocketfuel Naturals, chocolate haze. It has the right amount of everything that is quickly absorbed into my bloodstream and is amazingly filling without any crazy sugar and/or caffeine blood sugar rushes that can cause me to crash. They have other great flavors, and I highly suggest you try them one day.

Now if solid food or the thought of it makes you sick, try and figure out a smoothie recipe that offers protein and carbs but make sure you don't get all bogged down or put too much fiber in it. Sometimes soy products, or certain fruits, can cause upset tummy and you may spend the start of the race in the porto potty.

Consider almond butter as a "solid" mixed in, along with coconut water and maybe a scoop of a whey protein that you've already tested. Just don't go without some sort of fuel for breakfast.

Timing of your food is important and individualized. Decrease your food intake up to the race start. If you must, reach for something like half of a protein bar, half of a Pocketfuel Naturals packet, or a half or whole banana.

During
As I type I am training for the Maui to Molokai downwind race, 27 miles of open-ocean. I hope to finish in 4 +/- hours if all goes well. My challenge will be fluids. I have to think ahead and possibly wear two hydration packs. I'm not allowed to touch the boat. I may have an assistant jump in the water to hand me another hydration pack as another option for hydrating and eating.

I will only rely on Pocketfuel Naturals, chocolate haze. The convenient single packs are easy to carry in my hydration packs. This is what continues to work best for me. It worked for me when I did Molokai to Oahu. Why mess up a good thing?

Whether you're paddling two miles for pleasure or racing across a channel for thirty two, you must think about how to achieve simple, fast delivery of important nutrients to the body without ill effects such as bloating, nausea, or extreme sugar spikes that can cause you to crash. Your body is like your car—you need high-octane fuel that is long lasting and can be easily digested to turbo burst the engine.

Some of you may reach for gels, gummies or fig bars. Be careful of too much sugar. Think of time, ease of use, and how you can get this through healthy, real food. And heck yes, I'm going to plug again Pocketfuel Naturals because I really believe in it and bonus; there are lots of delicious flavors.

I will put a little bit of Heed electrolyte in my hydration pack. I use lemon lime flavor to help with hydration. I've had to really get this down to the bare minimum, as my stomach is super sensitive.

If there is the possibility of seasickness on a certain course you should also be prepared for that as well. It's happened to me before here on Maui in light wind and huge swell. It's awful.

The best thing you can do is start ingesting ginger a few days before if there is an anticipated swell or if you are going to be on a boat waiting for transitions. There are lots of great things you can eat that have ginger. I like ginger chews, (kept in a dry pouch) and ginger carbonated water sold in small cans which can be kept on the boat.

Not all of you will have huge endurance race days as your first race, but I wanted to mention this because one day you may have a channel crossing as your goal. Best to start thinking short and long-term and always have a plan B.

The general rule of thumb during a race is hydration first and food second if a longer distance or channel crossing. You've already read what to drink earlier in this chapter, now you have to decide or not to consider solids.

After
Victory! Well you've made it!

Whether it's three miles or 32, your body needs to get back to a normal state. While you may be tempted to throw down a cold one, best to wait and, if at all possible, completely pass until maybe the next day. Not to be boring, but having a recovery plan to help your body quickly switches gears into repair mode is and important part of being a successful SUP athlete. This is especially critical if you are racing the next day.

You can refer to the section earlier in this chapter to select the perfect recovery drink. Always be prepared to have it chilled and on hand.

As for food, best to keep it light and keep in mind our carb and protein needs. You'll want to eat something, but nothing to too crazy. I'll mention again, how great Pocketfuel Naturals is as a handy and quick recovery food right after hard training or after any length of race.

Portions are also important. Leave the temptation to pig out for another time, as your organs need to rest too. If you gorge yourself with too much food right after, I promise you will pay the price.

I remember after the M20 I was so happy because of how strong I felt at the finish. I couldn't believe it. Granted, I did relay, but considering I paddled across Hawaii's deepest channel and had been up since 4am and on a boat jumping off into big swells during transitions, I was pretty stoked with my nutrition planning and hydration for the race.

Some days are great like this and others will go the opposite way. The best thing you can do for yourself is to practice the art of recovery. If you do it enough times, and keep notes about what works best, your practice will serve you for many miles to come.

FACTORS AFFECTING A PADDLER'S NUTRITION NEEDS

Touring/travel

Many elite paddlers who tour and travel to different and exotic locations for SUP tournaments often find themselves struggling to maintain proper nutrition while away from the structure and convenience of home base. Some of you perhaps are just starting to think about traveling to an exciting racing destination? Either way, both types of paddlers need to consider travel as a factor that can interrupt or throw off your nutrition regime big time.

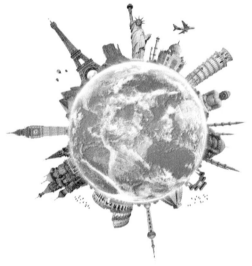

No matter where in the world you may travel to paddle, I have a few tips that can help you reduce the possibilities of eating challenges that could hinder your performance outcome.

Also, as your body enters a new time zone, two or more, your entire body's rhythm and functions need time to adjust and adapt. Even if you're traveling across just one time zone you, as a SUP athlete, may experience such physical and physiological problems including:

- Severe dehydration
- Diarrhea / constipation / headaches
- Fatigue
- Mental stress / mood changes / irritability
- Loss of appetite

The more time zones from home you're traveling, the earlier you should arrive so that you can adapt and adjust your body's rhythm. The more you travel the more you will learn about your own needs and how to adjust.

Additionally, if you know you are traveling to a super hot and humid or really dry or cold environment, prepare well and adjust your hydration needs accordingly. And don't forget altitude. Acclimating to thinner air also takes time. Try and get in some time on the water before your race in those conditions that are new for your body.

Lastly, in regards to travel, beware of international foreign germs and diseases. Nothing is worse than contracting some unusual virus. Traveling far already tends to wear down your immune system.

Study the location you are going to, or ask your doctor if he or she is aware of anything that can expose you to an unwanted bug. With that said, keep your immune system protected and strong and make sure you are up to date on any shots that are required. Wash your hands all the time and don't be embarrassed to wear a protective face mask on the plane or in really crowded areas. You just never know.

You may have your own traveling rituals that help you ease into the next time zone. Keep those in practice and maybe add a few of these too:

Tips for Recovering Quickly While Traveling
• Hydrate as much as possible while on plane and avoid alcohol and caffeine.
• Wash hands often and wipe down eating trays with bacterial wipes.
• Practice methods to help you sleep as much as needed on plane.
• Wear light or medium "graduated" compression stockings under pants to help improve circulation for super long plane rides. These can be full or below the knee with open toe. Ask your doctor.
• If you need a special meal, call airline in advance and ask for extra veggies to help with hydration and to avoid constipation.
• Suck on low sugar throat drops to avoid dry or irritated throat because a dry throat can catch bugs more easily.
• Consider nose saline spray to keep nasal passage clean and moist.
• Reduce jet lag by maintaining regular sleep. Try to stay up in that time zone and go to bed in your destination's time frame. Get on the local time as soon as possible.
• Rule of thumb per time zone: Allow one full day per zone to adapt and let your body catch up.
• Try and jump into your training and paddling routine as fast as possible.

How to eat on the road

The wheels have touched down and you're super stoked. Your board is also safe and your paddle is not busted into five pieces. All good. But now you've learned that your friend's aunt's neighbor's dog rancher is going to be late to pick you up. Like four hours late! You're starving and you could eat your slippers. You're tired and you can't see straight. The world is dark and you're tired, hungry, and want to rest. Your energy is starting to crash. Anxiety is creeping in.

But wait, you're good. You suddenly perk up like someone just handed you the winning jersey. In your carry on, deep in that side pocket, you've packed healthy snacks that you love and that your body loves and that will get you through. Hooray! Something you know and you quickly reach for it and enjoy each bite. No need to walk up to a street vendor that has "things" hanging off a cart with fruit (you think) that's all bruised and spoiled.

Tips to help you while eating and paddling on the road
• If you can't recognize it, don't eat it.
• Bring as many healthy snacks (grain bars, box of raisins) as you can possibly pack.
• Drink only bottled water; avoid tap or water in glasses.
• If you're really going deep in jungle or remote locals, include a pack of water purification tablets to avoid serious bacteria.
• Bring one box of soda crackers in case you end up with a bad stomach.
• If junk food is the only or safest option try and find pastas, baked potatoes, or hamburgers without the vegetables on them (that could be tainted). Minimize fried food or high-sugar food.

If you're traveling in familiar countries such as the United States, Canada, and Europe more than likely, you'll have a better time selecting healthy, safer foods that are pretty consistent to what you eat now. There are plenty of breads and pastas for sure. Always stick to bottled water when possible.

However if you are stuck in who knows where and you can't find anything safe to eat, stick to breads, hardboiled eggs for protein if possible, and avoid trying anything over the top. Stick to your plan and training strategies as best as possible. You've come all this way. Why ruin your chances of blowing up and out on race day?

MY SPIN ON SUPPLEMENTS

First and foremost don't believe anything you read or hear about nutrition if they are trying to sell you something and making crazy claims. If you think the old adage "it's too good to be true" applies, paddle away fast. Do your homework and always consult your physician especially if you are taking any prescription medications.

Unless you have a medical condition that requires you to take an extra vitamin or two, or you are low on iron or B12 or others, I'd stay away. Now, some of you may want to whack me with your paddle, and fine—go ahead—but I'll duck faster than you can sweep because my body is clean and simple and pure.

If you feel in your hearts that whatever you are taking is helping you and not harming you, then more power to you. There are *some* products that are nice and clean and I will always keep an open mind to explore new things.

As a trainer I've seen it all and heard it all. I've tested myself to see what these things are like and I have to say supplements are mostly a way to make others rich. Especially those crazy little high profit cans of energy boosters with the initials R and B (but no name will be mentioned) that help you leap off tall buildings in a single bound? Oh and how about those little bottles of "blank" hour energy you see on check out counters that have killed people. *Come on!*

I am VERY particular when it comes to eating real food versus trying to pop a pill. I DO believe that you can find high quality food in small packages. Take, for instance, Pocketfuel Naturals. I said it again. This is real food that comes in a fast and convenient package.

Another company I give lots of credit to is HAMMER products. Their research is science- and medical-based with real athletes. They take the time to really educate the consumer and don't hide behind their labels.

I also think that if you have certain food allergies or are vegetarian some products used to supplement the diet are okay. Smoothies with a base of healthy liquid such as coconut water or soy milk are usually fine when high quality protein powders with fruit or veggies added.

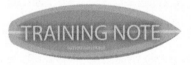 *Use common sense and try to eat real food for your SUP nutrition performance.*

EXAMPLES OF REAL FOOD FOR WINNING FUELING

In this section, I list ideas of what to eat so you can create healthy menus that fuel you. You are probably already familiar with many of these foots but simply need to be reminded of them. Below I have charts listing my favorite proteins, fats, and carbs that will help you make the best fueling choices.

Protein

Here are two examples of protein sources: animal (complete proteins – proteins that offer a good source of all the essential amino acids) and non animal (incomplete proteins – proteins that are missing some of the essential amino acids), but are still a good source of protein.

If you prefer not to eat animal proteins, you can combine two incomplete proteins to help fill in some of those essential amino acids. I do recommend organic and/or grass fed. See chart below:

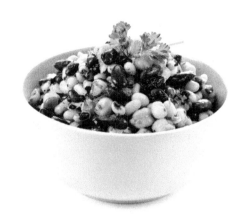

Complete Protein: Animal Proteins, Organic Preferred
Fish Chicken Pork Turkey Eggs Egg whites Bison Beef Cottage cheese Yogurt

Incomplete Proteins: Non-Animal, Organic Preferred		
Nuts	**Grains**	**Legumes**
Peanuts Pumpkin seeds Walnuts Almonds Cashews Sunflower seeds Sesame seeds Nut butters Peanut butter Almond butter	Quinoa Amaranth Barley Rolled oats Bulgur Rye Granola	Adzuki beans Chickpeas Black beans Garbanzo beans Kidney beans Lima beans Lentils Soy products Hummus Edamame

Combo Samples of Making Complete Proteins:
You can choose to use animal or non animal combinations: Yogurt with almonds   Bean and cheese burrito   Salad with kidney and lima beans and a hard boiled egg   Oatmeal with walnuts   Edamame dipped in hummus

Fats

Earlier in this chapter I talked about the importance of fat and how fat stores can contain more than 50 times the amount of energy contained in carbohydrate stores.

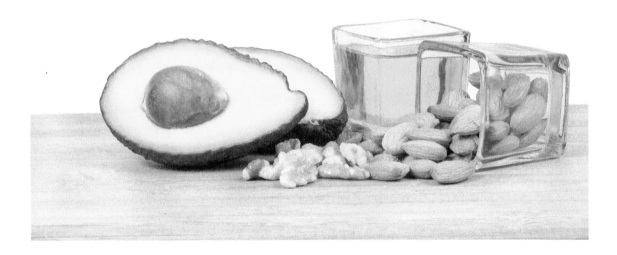

Healthy Fats This chart will include only Mono and Polyunsaturated Fats	
Monounsaturated Fats	Polyunsaturated Fats
Avocados Most nuts Olive, Sesame, Sunflower, Canola oil Olives Peanut butter	Safflower oil Margarine Fatty Fish – salmon, tuna Tofu Soy milk

Carbohydrates

As a reminder, carbs, especially complex carbs such as glucose, are the main sources of fuel so high quality choices matter. **Starch** is probably the most important energy source in an athlete's diet because it is broken down and stored as glycogen. For more information on this please refer to the section in this chapter called **A little science on nutrients as fuel**. Be careful not to select carb items that have too much fiber as they can cause bloating or upset stomach and gas.

Complex Carbs, Healthy Starches, and Whole Grains	
Brown rice	Sweet potato
Wild rice	Acorn squash
Quinoa	Spaghetti squash
Rolled oats	Butternut squash
Steel cut oats	Pumpkin
Amaranth	
Millet	
Sorghum	
Spelt	
Buckwheat	
Lentils	
Whole wheat pasta	

PRE RACE FUELING TIPS & COMPETITION WRAP UP

I imagine many of you have a lot of this under your rash guard pretty well, but let's just take a moment to review a few things as we close this chapter.

1. The BIGGEST suggestion in this chapter I can offer you is to never ever try anything new the day of your big SUP competition. I'm guilty and maybe you are too. Don't be tempted when your friend next to offers some weird looking gummy goo or squirt of this or that. This is why we train well in advance to test out the tummy and watch for any adverse signs that can lead disastrous results.

2. Prepare your own fuel. Make a clear list of exactly what you need and get it at least two weeks in advance. Although a boyfriend, girlfriend, or coach may know you well and has great intentions, it's best to be in charge of your own fate. Prepare in advance, and if traveling with extra stuff is an issue or hassle, ship your extra personal fuel needs to the location to which you're traveling and have the hotel or friends guard it with their lives.

3. There are many variables that can temporarily sideline the best SUP athlete's fueling game plan. The best leave their stubbornness at home and recognize the need to make small changes during an event if necessary, and also recognize that there will be some days that don't go right.

What I'm saying is: if your food and fuel plan is not working, be prepared to adjust so you don't completely sabotage your race and have to pull out. For example, some people think if they are working harder, and they are starting to crash harder the best reaction is to consume more calories. Sometime, actually, less is more. You don't always have to replace calorie for calorie. It's best to go light on the solid foods and focus on electrolyte replacement.

Go get'em!

References:

The Navy Seal Nutrition Guide

Peak Performance of Canada

Runners World

Journal of Athletic Training

(1) Human Kinetics: Expert from Sport Nutrition, Second Edition, by Asker Jeukendrup, PhD, and Michael Gleeson, PhD.

(2) Sports Hydration: '07

Originally presented as *Endurance Sports, Rehydration, Cerebral Edema and Death* at NEAFS (Northeastern Association of Forensic Scientists) Annual Meeting, Rye Brook NY, November 2, 2006 James Wesley M.S. Forensic Chemist, Clinical Toxicologist, Rochester, NY

(3) Livestrong What Are The Benefits of Baking Soda by Solomon Nwhator

(4) *Journal of Athletic Training* National Athletic Trainers' Association Position Statement: Fluid Replacement for Athletes

(5) Nancy Clark's Sports Nutrition Guidebook

CHAPTER 9
How to Create Your Own Winning SUP Training Program

- Defining and charting your paddling goals.
- Preparing and planning.
- Holding your course.
- Creating your own training program.
- FREE Paddling & Training Log download.
- Keeping your workouts fresh to avoid plateaus.
- Sample SUP strength training programs: from beginner to intermediate and pro levels.

You've been learning some good stuff. Now it's time to gather all of the information and put it into a action SUP plan. It's time for you to start thinking short and long term and begin training smarter. This is also a good time to start making sure that you always paddle with a purpose and record your efforts each and every time you hit the water. I wrote a good article about this if you'd like to take a quick peek. It's called **Making the Most of Your Paddling Sessions**. You can read it here: *http://bit.ly/1VxsOvv*

Once you've shaped some ideas and listed your goals you can develop your own personal training program to make sure you reach those goals. Because each of you is unique, you each need your own program. I believe that one program cannot fit all so I'll be sharing a couple of sample templates that will help you start building your own workout and training routine.

Here is an example of what a week of training might look like and things to think about:

Date/ Day	Time/ Session Length	Distance	Goals: Improve time, HR, technique, etc.	Results Time / Distance / Notes / Conditions / Rate Your Performance (1-10)
2/2/15 Monday	6AM / 45 mins	4-5 miles harbor	Increase cadence, paddle upwind	50 minutes, 5.5m, super windy choppy, 7 - Didn't feel 100%
	Studio			
2/5/15 Thursday	1PM / 1.5	8 miles Maliko	Downwinder, reduce HR, work on footwork	1 hr 20 min. HR Average 132, Lighter winds, 15-20, very onshore, Gotta get back more on fin faster, 9 - Felt good.
	Beach			
2/7/15 Saturday	7AM / ?	5 miles flat water Kihei	Cardio, better attitude about flat-water training!	**We'll see!**

Remember I'm always available to help you customize your program via SKYPE or when you come to Maui. Contact me via my website *SuzieTrainsMaui.com* to schedule an appointment.

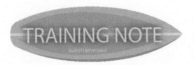

I have also created a FREE Paddling Training Log to help you track your goals and results. Download it here: http://bit.ly/1JCmgX8

DEFINING & CHARTING YOUR PADDLING GOALS

Remember in Chapter 7, The Mental Part, where I talk about defining the "why?" That's when you identify the goal or statement of the "why" and then begin put this programming into play. If you want to be successful in anything you seek to do you need to have a vision and a plan and the answer to the "why."

The why can be personal or it can because your sponsor expects you and you want to win the gold. The sooner you become crystal clear and cut to the chase, remove all obstacles and turn your laser focus beam to high, the faster you'll get over the finish line. An example "why" might be that you want to enter all of the local races this season.

This is where your fingers will hit the keyboard or, better yet, you can pull out a table and feel yourself write it down in the old fashioned way. Let your pen flow while you write down your thoughts and your biggest SUP dreams. You want to come to Maui and do a Maliko downwinder? Write it down. You want to do the Molokai to Oahu channel crossing? Write that down. You may think its nuts, but you'd be surprised at how your subconscious holds data. Before you know it, one day there you will be.

Let me help you start thinking about what you'd like to do with your paddling strength. The following example is, of course, trying to get you to Maui! Take a look. Keep it simple. This is just one example of what your year or couple of years out may look like. You have to start somewhere. Just start.

	Winner Will's Paddle Goals 2016		
Race	**Why**	**Distance**	**When:**
Saturday SUP Series Local Races Local SUP Club	For fun, training, social	5 miles	Every Saturday when time permits
Go to Maui to train with Suzie	Downwind paddling skills, SUP fitness strength training, learn ocean skills, build ocean endurance/ confidence	36-44 Miles	June, 1-2 weeks
Figure 8 Fun Course Ocean	New challenge, fun	8 miles	July
Gorge Downwind Race	Love downwind racing	13 miles	August
Future Goals			
OluKai Downwind race	Paddle with the best on Maui	8 miles	May
IMUA Paddle	Great cause, fun!	10 miles	Weekend after Olukai
Maui to Molokai	Personal goal Relay then solo one day	27	July

If you're pro level, your chart will be 3 times as long with lots races and events. Pick and choose wisely to avoid burnout and possible injury. Sometimes a cancellation is a blessing in disguise.

PREPARING AND PLANNING

I'm talking about everything from financial concerns, days off work, training, getting the right gear and executing your mission, and preparing your food. Your whole life, really.

My clients who are most successful have a great approach to this and allow me to help them make it real and realistic. When you start doing the math and think of cost and time involved, you may need to adjust a few races or maybe move one to the next year.

You might also discover along the way that you might not be ready for one particular race or two. Make peace now with the idea of that potentially happening. It's okay.

Next do an inventory of your paddling equipment and your training equipment. Make sure you have the right stuff in all departments to help you do your best. But don't break the bank! Make sure you can keep food in your refrigerator.

In addition to the boards and paddle equipment, if you want to train to win, you have to make sure that you have all of the proper training gear (or belong to a gym that has the gear). I've presented exercises that are simple and require just the basic type of training equipment. Most gyms will have everything except for maybe the Indo Board gear and the half foam roller.

The most important thing as you are now thinking like that athlete you are from Chapter 7 is to keep your fuel feeding the SUP machine (which is you). When you prepare and shop, always include your eating program as part of your SUP training program.

I would expect by now you could train me! The food is key so don't skimp on that if possible. Eating healthy doesn't have to be expensive. Do your research on who has the best prices. I know I wish we had a Trader Joe's here on Maui instead of that store we call Whole Paychecks.

HOLDING YOUR COURSE

When I say this, I mean to say, "Expect the unexpected in life and hold out your really big catcher's mitt, because now and then life will throw you a really hard screw ball." You have to catch it, examine it and find a way to deal with it as best you can. It may mean the need to postpone a race or two, but whatever the matter, take care of your total well-being first.

If a couple of wheels fall off the wagon in your life for a little while or for a short time, that's okay. That can actually make you a tougher paddler, mentally. If you are paddling along in life in a plastic bubble and are never faced with challenges or diversity you're less likely to adapt to changes on the race course as well.

Welcome change or hard times; pull up your board shorts or bikini bottoms and take care of matters where you're needed most. Paddling is always there for you and so are those who support you.

All joking aside, hold your course in life so that you can hold your course come race day. Some of the best paddlers I know have ups and downs in their lives. Things aren't always as they appear, especially on social media!

Allow for changes and expect them but remember how happy paddling makes you and you'll always have that to look forward to.

Creating Your Own Training Program

Now on to the nitty gritty. You have lots of tools in your toolbox from this book and it's up to you how you use them. I would like you to put on your trainer hat and start thinking how you will approach an actual training session. I will now help you formulate a program that offers you all the benefits of what you've read so far and make it come to life.

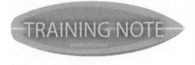

Along with all of the land training you'll be doing from the help of my book, I wanted you to also incorporate the use of my FREE Paddling Training Log. This is an additional tool to help you reach your "why" and your goals. Download it here: http://bit.ly/1JCmgX8

The best thing you can do for yourself and for your paddling is to always mix it up with every session. Keep your goals in mind but also allow and give yourself some variety so you don't get stale or plateau.

There is no perfect, or "right" program that will fit all but the following tips will definitely help you.

What every workout should include: (assuming the workout is one hour and does not include cardio)

- Warm Up: 5 minutes
- Core Exercises: 1-4 of your choice with progressions
- Balance Work: 2-4 various progressions
- Strength: 1 exercise for each muscle group
- ABS: 1-2 different exercises
- Cool Down: 5 minutes

The **warm up** can be anything that gets your body moving. It could be high knee marches, easy gentle fast moving small squats, easy groovy ice skaters side to side, swimming circles with alternating arms in both forward and/or back motions, ten split lunges forward and back, 5-10 light kettle bell swings. Just nothing static—meaning a stretch you'd hold in one position. Get that body moving.

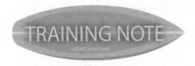

For the warm up, I'd rather you use your own body weight instead of a treadmill, elliptical or stationary bike.

Core Exercises you can select some good ones from Chapter 2. Just choose one to three exercises and do one or two sets of 10-12 reps. Don't overkill on the core. The core needs to warm up first before you stress your body in other ways. Try some progressions along the way for added challenge.

Your **balance work** can be two to three different platforms or two to three exercises using the same piece of equipment. You can choose. Play with your progressions safely. Refer to Chapter 3 or go to my website for lots of exercise samples and more.

The **strength** component of your training can include many different things, depending upon how much time in the week you have to train. For example, if I am training 3 times in my studio and 3 days on the water my strength training might look like this:

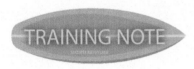 *This is just focusing on the strength part. You will always do core and balance with each workout session. The samples below are pretty heavy weeks. You can always adjust accordingly.*

Sample One:

Monday:	**Total Body Training** – Every Muscle Group (1) Exercise 1-3 sets
Tuesday	Paddle 1 hour + 30 min cardio
Wednesday	**Lower Body** - 2-3 different exercises Legs, Hamstrings
Thursday	Paddle 1 hour + 30 min cardio
Friday	**Upper Body** - 2-3 different exercises Shoulders, Chest, Upper Back
Saturday	Maliko Run 8 -10 Miles
Sunday	Rest

Sample Two:

Monday:	**Total Body Training** – Every Muscle Group (1-2) Exercise 1-3 sets
Tuesday	Paddle 1 hour + Tabata
Wednesday	**Total Body Training** – Every Muscle Group (1-2) Exercise 1-3 sets
Thursday	Paddle 1 hour + 30 min cardio
Friday	**Total Body Training** – Every Muscle Group (1-2) Exercise 1-3 sets
Saturday	Paddle Surfing 1.5 hrs
Sunday	Rest

I always tell my clients to do your **abs** last. Sorry, your core work does not count. We do our abs absolutely last because they work all throughout your workout to hold you up and help you execute each exercise.

Your **cool down** can be as easy as a quick self myofascial roll out, a few stretches on the stability ball or even a chill walk. Keep your cool down simple and drink plenty of water.

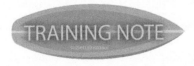
Over the years theories and opinions change about when to "stretch" all your muscles. This event is actually It's own mini training session and best done in the evening before you go to sleep. Holding a static stretch for more than 30 seconds signals the body it's time to go to sleep. When we do this mid day or in the morning it confuses the body and the benefit is not as great.

AVOIDING PLATEAUS BY INTRODUCING VARIABLES TO KEEP YOUR WORKOUTS FRESH

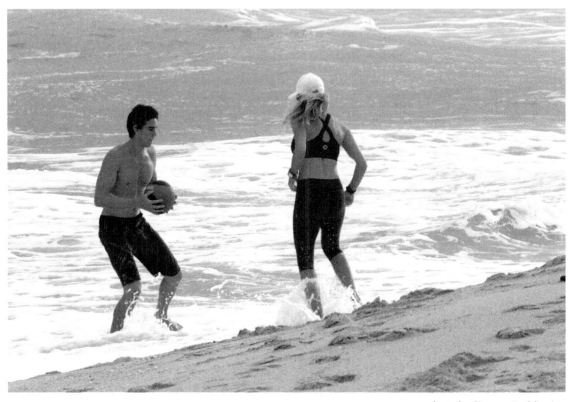

photo by Simone Reddingius

A fun workout will keep you motivated and inspired. But more importantly, if you don't vary your workouts, your body will actually get bored actually before your mind does and it will stop changing at a certain point. (Which means your progress will slow or stop.) This is true for training in general. If you don't introduce change you will stop winning. You may like routine but I guarantee your body needs new fresh ways to train.

When I'm helping clients reach their goals and avoid plateaus, I am forever and always changing up their routines on the fly. Half the time they don't even know I'm doing it! I've gotten pretty good at it and the results show!

There are many ways you can change the training variables, such as changing intensity levels, varying your speed and tempo, adding more or less weight and so on and so forth. Never ever get complacent in your workouts.

EXAMPLES OF HOW YOU CAN CHANGE UP THE VARIABLES FOR YOUR SUP TRAINING PROGRAM

- Strength train in a circuit style with little to no rest. Move quickly between exercises.
- Train at the beach or outside at a park.
- Alternate balance exercise—first on two feet, the next set on one foot.
- Switch between interval paddling sprints and slow and steady pacing.
- Add a small set of plyometrics in between each strength set.
- Start with heavy weights and finish with lighter weights, then reverse the order during the next session.
- Change the platform on which you are training. For example do one set of bicep curls standing on BOSU and one set standing on the Indo Board Gigante Cushion.
- Do A BOP style of training: A few paddle laps and then back to the beach for some push ups.
- Perform one set at a fast tempo, followed by a set at a more medium-paced tempo.
- Select a super challenging leg exercise, followed by a less difficult set.
- Add an extra one to three second hold on a rep.
- Add an extra set to each muscle group.
- Add five more reps to the last set.
- For endurance, do more reps with less weight or resistance.

Sample SUP Strength Training Program Templates

I've created a couple of sample SUP Strength Training Program Templates for you to try. Please keep in mind you must use caution and common sense when creating a program for yourself, as only you know your current level of fitness. So the first one is for beginner to intermediate level SUP Athletes and the other is for the Pros.

Just a reminder—remember that your paddling programs are completely separate from your SUP strength training programs. The following exercises can be found in previous chapters. I have a million and one combinations of how I could have put together this paddling program but each exercise has the paddler's functional strength in mind.

Sample One:

Beginner – Intermediate Level Paddler
5 Minute Warm up: (10) Alternating side lunges, (10) trunk twists, (10) active inner thigh stretches, (10) 5-8 pound kettlebell or dumbbell swings (10) Alternating forward swimming strokes (10) High marches in place. Repeat.

CORE Exercises	Sets	Reps or time	Intensity	Tempo	Rest
Prone floor plank Progress to 1 leg	2	15-30s	Controlled	Slow	15s
Stability ball kneeling	2-3	30s-45s	Calm control	Slow	
BOSU sitting Add 8lb dumbbell moving left and then to right side	2-3	12-15	Controlled & smooth	Slow with 1-2s holds	10 15s
BALANCE Exercises					
1 leg all planes of motion on ½ foam roller	2	5 each leg	Lose upper body	Medium	None
1 leg all planes of motion on Indo Board Gigante Cushion & on Kicktail	2	5 each leg	Lose upper body, controlled	Medium	None
Surf stance squats goofy foot & regular Indo Board + Gigante Cushion	2	10	Lose upper body	Medium with 1-2s hold	None

Strength	Exercises	Sets	Reps	Intensity	Rest
SHOULDER	Standing prone paddling tube Presses	1-3	12-15	Controlled	30s
BACK	Stability ball seated tube rows	1-3	12-15	Smooth with 2-3s hold	30s
CHEST	1 arm on BOSU 1 arm on ground push ups knee bent or full	1-3	10 r/l	Controlled and good breathing	1 min+
LEGS	Alternating walking lunges 8-15 pounds	1-3	24-30	Smooth	1 min+
BICEPS	Standing 2 arm curls 8-10 pounds add BOSU last set	1-2	12-15	Controlled, light grip	30s
TRICEPS	Standing tube press downs	1-2	12-15	Controlled with 2s hold	30s
ABS	Chest lifts	1	25-75	Steady breath	None

Sample Two:

Elite Pro Level Paddler
5 Minute Warm Up: (10) Forward split lunges, (10) trunk twists, (10) active inner thigh stretches with medicine ball, (10) 10 pound kettlebell swings (10) Alternating forward and backward swimming strokes, repeat

CORE Exercises	Sets	Reps or time	Intensity	Tempo	Rest
Advanced 1 legged plank with feet on BOSU	2	30s ea leg	Controlled	Slow	30s
Stability ball kneeling with 8lbs medicine ball in and outs	2	12-15	Smooth & controlled	Medium	30s
! Knee BOSU kneeling with 8 pound medicine ball moving leg in all planes of motion	2	5 each leg	Smooth & controlled	Slow with 1-2s holds	30-45s

BALANCE Exercises					
Half foam roller single leg touchdowns w/8 pound dumbbell	2	5 each leg	Smooth & controlled	Medium	30s
Paddle board atop of fully inflated Gigante Cushion regular/goofy stance	2	Each direction 30s -1min	Smooth & controlled	Slow	45s
BOSU to BOSU forward hops with a twist	2	10	Lose upper body	Medium with soft landing	45s
BOSU to BOSU singles side to side	2	25 total	Controlled	Medium to Fast	15-30s

Strength	Exercises	Sets	Reps	Intensity	Rest
SHOULDER	Tube chops one set on ground then on BOSU	2-3	12-15	Smooth & controlled	30s
BACK	TRX RIP TRAINER back rows	2-3	12-15	Smooth with 2-hold	30s
CHEST	TRX RIP TRAINER chest presses	2-3	12-15	Controlled and good breathing	1 min+
LEGS	Squats on Gigante Flo Cushion with 15 pound kettlebell	2-3	12-15	Smooth steady+ 2s hold	1 min+
BICEPS	Seated alternation regular curls 8-15+ not too heavy	2-3	24-30	Controlled, light grip	30s
TRICEPS	Bench dips 1 regular set Other 1 foot on BOSU	2-3	12-15	Controlled with 2s hold	30s
ABS	Chest lifts		75-200	Steady breath	None

You can tweak all of the above programs. You can start at the shoulders and do circuit style one group after the next and repeat to the top. You can also select exercises that are completely without or with weights.

You can also add a splash of cardio exercises between each set if you want to train at an elevated heart rate. For example you could perform ten jumping jacks after each strength set or five burpees. I like to have my clients perform 5-10 BOSU hop ups with two feet between EACH set. Eventually that will equal almost 100 reps and the benefit is huge.

Before I close this chapter I want to add a few more tips and reminders to make sure you have the best workouts ever and win more races.

OTHER SUP PROGRAM TRAINING TIPS

- If you find yourself pooping out midway through your workout, stop and regroup and maybe hit the reset button by going for a quick two minute walk outside. Take a bite of something you can easily digest. Clear your head and then gauge your energy for the remainder of your workout.

- When training remember to preserve your energy and training sessions from water to land. Don't overload your training so that by day four you are too spent. And, by all means, take a day off if you really need to. That can really help. Rest and recharge.

- If you start your workout in a crappy mood or if you're emotionally distracted, hopefully your mood will change and get better as you go. Monitor yourself and make sure that it's "the right" time to train. Be there 100% or go do something else. These are the times you can make dumb training moves and get injured.

- When in doubt about whether or not to push yourself to the next level maybe go at 50% and work your way up from there. Proper form and technique is critical to a successful day on water. You can always have me sit in with you on a SKYPE session or two. It's a blast and it's really effective.

- And lastly, some days you will just have "those days" and that's part of growing and learning how to adapt as a paddling pro. You have to go with the flow and even when your mind says go and body says no, your body wins. Take it easy.

I hope you found this chapter to be helpful. Remember to refer back to the earlier chapters for tons of exercises you can progress with. And be sure to check out more training tips and videos at *SuzieTrainsMaui.com*

CHAPTER 10
Common Overuse Injuries Related SUP

- Some of the most common injuries related to SUP.
- Muscle Groups and their associated injuries.
- Recovery: the importance of rest.

It's well known that SUP requires muscles and nerves in the entire body to perform and respond in unison. You're never isolating one muscle group at any given moment. For example, as you paddle, your entire shoulder complex, upper/lower back, feet, ankles, knees, hips, and core (everything excluding your extremities) are executing each short or long stroke in a smooth, connected fashion.

If any part of that kinetic chain is not greased, strong, or well tuned, your stroke will fall short. What often happens when we paddle while nursing a nagging particular injury, is that other parts of your body may also get weak which can cause you to set yourself up for an additional unwanted injury. Read this section to learn all how you can best avoid this from occurring.

Whether you paddle on the weekends or 5 days a week as a professional, most of you will eventually experience an injury—if you haven't already. It's not surprising, considering the sheer number of people entering the sport, that there are many paddlers who encounter one or two possible nagging, temporary, or long-term set backs.

This chapter is not meant as a diagnostic tool. I am not a physician and I always suggest you consult with a specialist for any specific concerns.

COMMON AREAS OF INJURY

As you may have guessed, the **shoulder** is the most common area of injuries and strains, in addition to **biceps tendons, lower back, upper back,** and the external area of the **elbow**. Others have also reported problems with the exterior part and outside of the **knee**.

While it's true that those areas mentioned above are the most commonly affected, because of all of the different styles and race disciplines evolving there will always be other areas of injury. These could include possible broken ribs from white water or SUP-cross and more serious injuries such as fin lacerations, shoulder separations, and concussions from big wave wipeouts.

The more you know about how each muscle works with regards to paddling the better you'll be able to approach your land and water training. The end result will be a stronger SUP performance with each stroke and a stronger, injury-free body.

SHOULDER

The shoulder complex is more complicated than one might assume. It's where the power from your core gets transferred to the paddle blade, and finally to the water. Don't for a minute underestimate the importance of training the shoulder in a consistent, balanced manner. If your shoulders fail, you'll be stuck on the beach for a bit, or at least skimming the top of the water with your paddle for a while until you're healed and strong again.

You may have heard of the group of muscles called the rotator cuff muscles.

Rotator Cuff Muscles

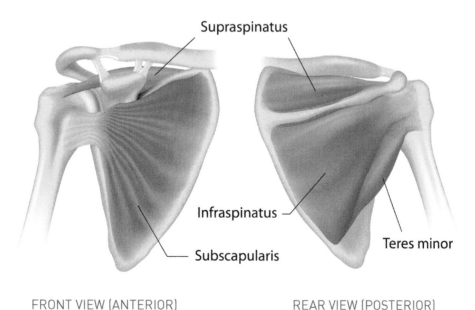

Supraspinatus

Infraspinatus

Subscapularis

Teres minor

FRONT VIEW (ANTERIOR)   REAR VIEW (POSTERIOR)

The paddle stroke is a combination of medial rotation and abduction (of the top hand). The deeper rotator cuff muscles included are the supraspinatus, subscapularis, infraspinatus and the teres minor. This requires the work of the subscapularis, latissimus dorsi, pec. minor, pec. major, and teres major along with deltoid and supraspinatus to lift the arm up.

The bottom hand acts mostly to stabilize while transferring the rotation of the trunk to the paddle. The muscles used to stabilize are mainly latissimus dorsi rhomboids, triceps, and middle fibers of the traps.

The rotator cuff muscles dynamically work in unison with each and every stroke. If one in the group is out of line, undertrained or over trained compensations may begin to set in, leading to weakness. Some will take more load and strain, leading to a possible worse case scenario—a tear. If you're going all out in a sprint on one side for over 30 minutes with no break, or you hit a wave with your paddle at a funny angle, you have a high risk for an injury to the shoulder.

Reported issues and injuries:

- Shoulder separation
- Numbing in the hands/fingers due to possible impingement patterns
- Weakness, soreness and/or pain at the joint and at the points of the supraspinatus and the infraspinatus from repetitive motion
- Partial or full tears due to impact injuries from big wave wipeouts or overuse
- Painful, radiating and/or shooting pain due to possible over training or undertraining of supporting upper back muscles and deeper rotator cuff muscles

One thing you can do is to be sure your paddle blade is not too wide. You'd be surprised what a drastic difference a narrow blade can offer, without causing you to lose power. Also make sure your stroke technique is not the culprit. Hire a pro to help you fine-tune your stroke. Also, refer back to Chapter 2 to learn how to get more power from your core to lessen the strain on your shoulders.

BICEPS TENDON

When we think of the bicep some of us may not realize there is an "s" at the end of the word biceps. The muscle is actually two long, strong tendons called the short head and the long head that work together as one. The tendons that connect the biceps to the top of the shoulder joint are called the proximal biceps tendons. The tendon that attaches the biceps muscle to the forearm bones (radius and ulna) is called the distal biceps tendon. The function of the biceps is to lift the arm up and outward.

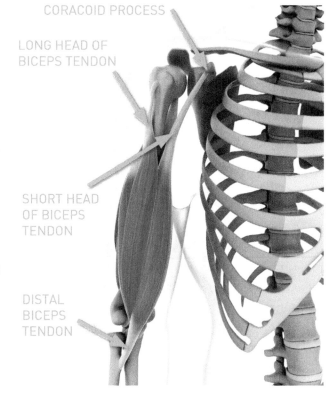

CORACOID PROCESS

LONG HEAD OF BICEPS TENDON

SHORT HEAD OF BICEPS TENDON

DISTAL BICEPS TENDON

In stand up paddling the biceps muscles and tendons are constantly under tension and are contracting with each stroke as you reach with the arm extended. This tension relationship from the shoulder joint all the way to your hand, and ultimately to the top of the paddle also risks the condition called bicep tendonitis. Bicep tendonitis is often caused by degeneration of the long head of the bicep tendon and/or can be aggravated with repetitive paddling motions—for instance, the shoulder lifting the paddle out of the water to initiate each stroke. Think of how many strokes we grind out per minute!

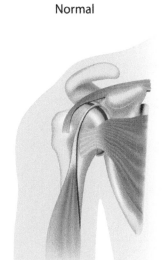

Normal

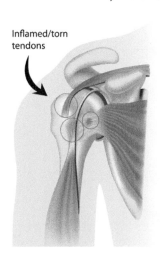

Rotator cuff problems

Inflamed/torn tendons

Sometimes this tendon gets inflamed, particularly when one tries to lift the arm up as if to lift the paddle or, in another example, to brush your hair. The pain can be deep and is sometimes reported as a throbbing pain in the front of the shoulder. In some cases the area may be tender to the touch. You may want to lighten your grip on the shaft and handle of paddle and see if that helps. Also check out the different diameter shafts and also consider a more flexible shaft.

Treatment for this is usually conservative with ice, rest, physical therapy sometimes PRP, or cortisone injections. Always consult your physician.

LOWER BACK

It's no wonder one's lower back may get sore, tired, or even strained with all the twisting and continuous bent over positions in which we find ourselves while "reaching" for the ultimate stroke. Often my lower back gets a little sore during distance paddling or when I'm paddling in side wind for longer stretches than normal.

When I watch some of the top paddlers' styles of really choking down the paddle shaft I can see the docs just lining up ready to offer care and advice. I get lots of emails from guys and gals who don't realize that by not having a strong core their lower back can suffer terribly when doing this.

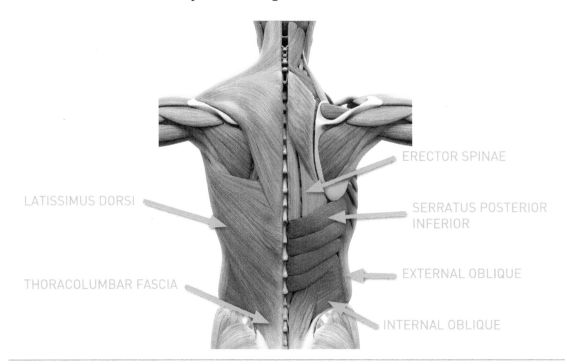

The lower back is part of our core and acts to stabilize and assist during every stroke. If this hurts then it's really hard to focus and paddle on.

I've been plagued by intense lower back injuries from dirt biking and windsurfing since I was 16. My injuries have been bad enough that I've had what is called "dropped leg syndrome" where the foot just gives out when it wants to without warning from the sciatic nerve being pinched at a lower level disc. It's a real drag. I've had such serious back injuries that I've needed surgical intervention. Some days I think it's a wonder I'm even walking. I'll have more on how to strengthen your back later in this chapter.

Some of the complaints I've heard and read of the lower back pain people experience as a result of stand up paddling are:

- Muscle spasms
- Intense seizing up of the low back
- Minor to major aches at one of the disc levels above the pelvic bone right or left side
- Radiating pain down the back of the leg and butt
- Bulged discs
- Pinched nerves

DISC PROBLEMS

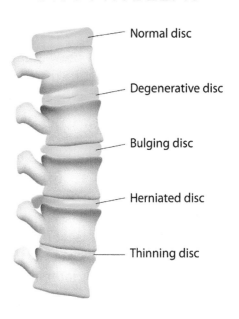

Normal disc

Degenerative disc

Bulging disc

Herniated disc

Thinning disc

Low back pains and strains are nothing to take lightly, regardless of age. Speaking of age, I hate to say it kids, but mild to moderate or severe disc degeneration can be due to natural wear and tear as a result of aging.

Most folks do fine with rest, ice, and/or heat. If you really think you did a number on yourself, especially if you felt a pop, if you were suddenly brought down to your knees, or if, at anytime, you are not getting better, please consult your physician. Sometimes rest and a little physical therapy can do wonders. I will cover how to strengthen your lower back and its supportive muscles so you can avoid common lower back strains during SUP.

You can also consider a paddle adjustment for the back like we talked about for the shoulder. If your paddle is too short your lower back may really suffer. I've also seen the reverse. If your paddle is too long you could possibly aggravate the upper trapezius and/or rhomboid region. For downwind paddling my paddle is a bit longer than my paddle surfing paddle. It's worth getting a proper fit and experimenting.

UPPER BACK

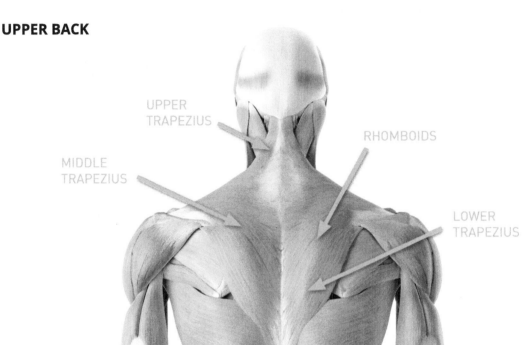

The upper back is often under stress as it's got a big job to hold up your head and upper torso, help your chest to breathe in and out, assist in maintaining your posture, and also help stabilize both shoulders as you paddle from side to side. The muscles of the upper back include the trapezius (upper, middle, lower), rhomboid major, and levator scapulae muscles, which anchor the scapula (shoulder blade) and clavicle to the spines of several vertebrae, as well as to the occipital bone of the skull.

I can't tell you how many people point to the back of their right or left shoulder and tell, me "right" there. They are often referring to that spot on the back of your shoulder blade that is super tender after they paddle. Or I'll have people tell me their traps get really sore after distance races. I can vouch for that. Mine tend to rise up to my ears, it seems, at mile number 18.

Again, look for the tips later in this chapter that will help you keep a healthy and pain-free upper back.

ELBOW

This has been an increasing area of complaints for many paddlers. So much so that I'm hearing it to be called "paddlers elbow." You've heard of tennis elbow? It's sort of the same thing. This is a super common overuse injury from stand up paddling.

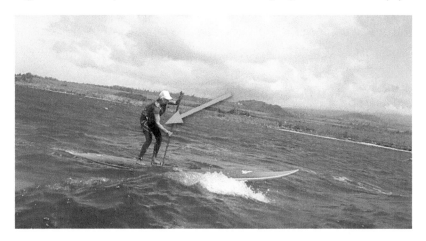

You'll notice that no matter how hard we try to remember not to overgrip or grab the shaft of the paddle too tightly with our lower hand, it's hard sometimes to me mindful of this in the heat of the moment—especially while you are grinding hard against wind.

The muscles and tendons in your forearm that help you extend your arm also open your wrist and fingers to allow the blade to enter the water. Then they have to pull and rotate the shaft back toward you to complete each stroke. They can really suffer from this repetitive pattern. That's a lot of gripping and wear and tear on those muscles.

The muscles and tendons in your forearm that insert to the outer or lateral portion of your arm and elbow and allow you to grip the paddle shaft are called extensors. These extensors attach the muscles to the bone and attach to what is called the lateral epicondyle.

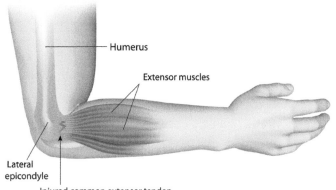

Humerus

Extensor muscles

Lateral epicondyle

Injured common extensor tendon

This tendon can be tender to touch and feel very weak at times. That tendon is called the Extensor Carpi Radialis Brevis. I have this problem on occasion and just have to do my stretches and be disciplined with icing and friction icing. Friction icing is like a form of deep massage and is a common method used by physical therapists. I will take 5 or so small Dixie cups and fill with water and freeze them. Then I rub them firmly on the outside of my elbow where it's tender. Not too hard. I highly suggest that you consult with your sports physician or physical therapist to make sure this is the best protocol for you.

Some people wear the compression bands you can buy at the drugstore to help prevent the tendons from rolling over each other, but I find them to cause more discomfort than help. And, as always, please consult your physician if you have problems.

I will show you a great stretch later in the chapter that can prevent or reverse this common SUP injury.

KNEE

The final overuse injury in SUP that I'll mention here is one that involves the outer area of the knee and is often referred to as Iliotibial band (ITB) syndrome. It feels like a dull ache and can be painful. It can also be seen in runners, surfers and hikers.

People have mentioned to me that they've experienced this pain while distance paddling. It's known that one of the causes of this is weak hip abductor muscles. These weak hip abductors (outer part of upper thigh) are part of a commonly seen pattern of weak core muscles. This leads to a muscle imbalance.

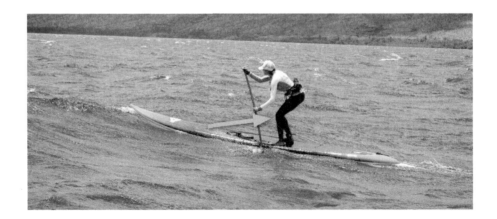

If you are just starting to increase the length or distance of your training sessions, your hip abductors can become fatigued and require the added assistance of the muscles that attach into the ITB to work harder.

The iliotibial band runs along the lateral or outside aspect of the thigh and is an important structure that stabilizes the outside of the knee as it flexes and extends. This is a thick band of muscles. Inflammation of the IT band can occur as it crosses back and forth across the bony prominence of the femoral epicondyle as the knee flexes and extends.

A good friend of mine, Clay Everline, MD, who is a surfer and paddler on Oahu and sees this often in his clinic wrote an article on this topic for Suzie Trains Maui. He said, "ITB syndrome can be problematic. The discomfort may be so intense as to discourage you from participating in the often long and rewarding sessions of SUP and other endeavors."

He also adds, "Ice massage is one of the best initial therapies for ITB syndrome. Hold a cube of ice in a napkin and massage the inflamed area until the cube has melted. It could take up to 20 minutes. Do this one or two times daily. A Cho-Pat strap or similar compression tape may prevent overstretching and inflammation, but ultimately it comes down to adjusting biomechanics and muscle balance."

Clay also mentions that surgery is rarely necessary. There are some great stretches and exercises below that show how you can prevent this injury from happening to you.

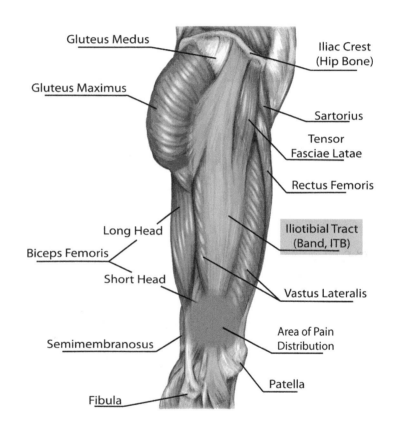

EXERCISES AND TRAINING TIPS TO STRENGTHEN THE SHOULDER FOR STAND UP PADDLERS

It's pretty amazing that, stroke after stroke, we can do what we do with such force, when you think of all of the shoulder muscles that must perform together at one time. To be consistently strong, each muscle needs the other to be on board. If one or two are weak or under or over trained, your stroke and SUP performance will suffer.

In the picture below I included an image of the chest along with the shoulder illustration to show how the chest acts as a major player and a strong stabilizing component.

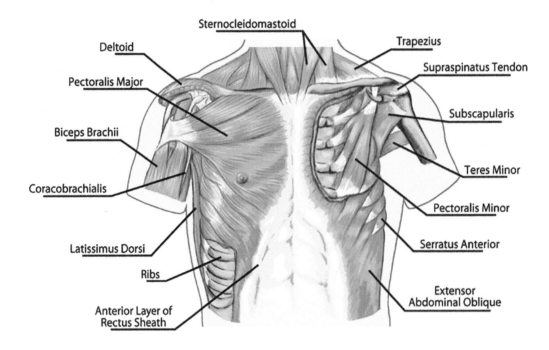

In this section I will give you my best exercises to help you maintain great shoulder health—specifically to help you avoid injury and keep your muscles in balance. You can also refer back to Chapter 4, **How to Increase Your Upper Body Strength & Endurance for SUP**

You can also check out some of the exercises I'll be sharing with you by watching my video called: **Stand Up Paddling Exercises to Increase Performance and Recovery Video With Suzie Cooney** here: *http://bit.ly/1Q9KCtO*

Exercise 1:
HOLD THE MONEY

Good posture is everything. A paddler's posture is always going to be challenged during daily life as the chest pectoral walls like to pull forward and create a sort of concave protraction. I've coined the term, "hold the money" for this exercise, which means to squeeze and pinch your shoulder blades together as if you're holding a $100 bill and you must not ever let go. It's also called retraction of the shoulder blades.

The muscles of the upper back work hard all throughout each stroke, especially when you're racing. It's easy to get fatigued and tired and very sore. A possible result of this fatigue is when you notice your head jutting forward, as the muscles of your neck, scalenes, will sometimes try and help, resulting in them becoming strained.

It's extra important to always work on your posture to increase your stand up paddling performance.

SUGGESTED TRAINING EQUIPMENT
None

SUGGESTED REPS/SETS
All day long!

PROGRESSION VARIABLES
None

Stand up nice and tall, neck relaxed, tilt your pelvis forward, roll your shoulders back and keep the chest out, all while you gently squeeze your shoulder blades together. That's how you roll from now on. (See picture on next page.)

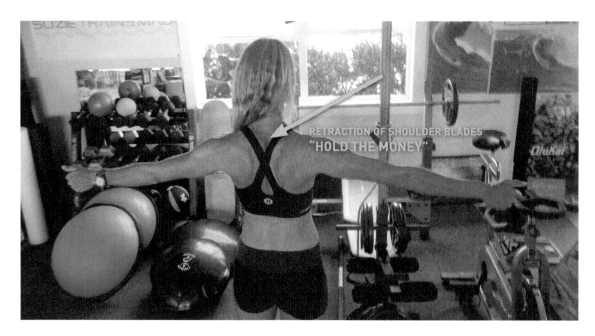

Exercise 2:
STANDING INTERNAL / EXTERNAL SHOULDER TUBE ROTATIONS

I will first start by saying this exercise is not the most exciting and, just like anything, practice makes you stronger. I feel it's the *second* most important one after the first exercise. So please make sure you add this one to your training regime as well.

SUGGESTED TRAINING EQUIPMENT
Light to medium gauge resistance tubing (I prefer ones with cushioned handle,) or cable with horseshoe handle, lighter weight setting

SUGGESTED REPS/SETS
15-20 each side, 1-2 sets

MOVEMENT TEMPO/SPEED
Controlled and smooth

PROGRESSION VARIABLES
Possibly heavier gauge tubing, but for this exercise more reps with lower resistance is best

PROGRESSION 1

Internal Tube Rotations (right shoulder)

Affix resistance tubing to a sturdy pole about waist high. Stand next to the pole so the pole is to your left and your right hand is holding tube handle. Your elbow should be tucked to your side and your arm bent at a 90 degree angle. Allow enough resistance to have some tension but not too much. This is your start position.

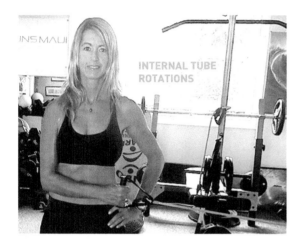 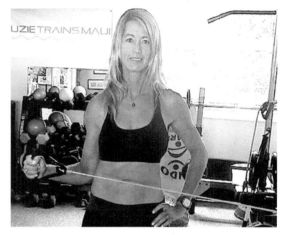

Next, with nice posture, pull the handle inside across your mid section while always keeping your shoulder blades gently pinched together. Then return to start position. Repeat the desired number of reps/sets.

PROGRESSION 2

External Tube Rotations (left shoulder)

Now switch to the left hand and begin with handle on outside of your hip and waist. With shoulders in gentle retraction or squeezed, pull handle towards center of body.

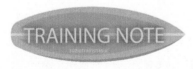

What's cool is simply to turn your body 180 degrees and do exactly the same on opposite side arms. Confused? You'll get it! Also don't make the tubing too taught. It should be a nice and smooth effort with excellent form for each rep.

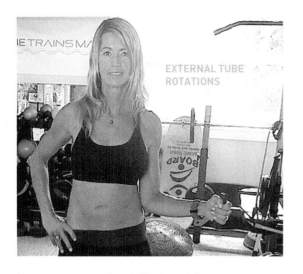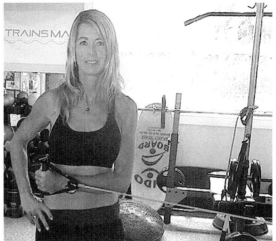

Repeat same for left shoulder.

Exercise 3:
STANDING SCAPTION RAISES

This is another must-do to help strengthen the muscles of the shoulder blades and supraspinatus while also strengthening the traps and rhomboids. This is also great to help you improve your posture and build upper body endurance. You'll really feel these the next day!

SUGGESTED TRAINING EQUIPMENT
Light weights—2-5 pounds

SUGGESTED REPS/SETS
12-15 each side, 1-2 sets

MOVEMENT TEMPO/SPEED
Controlled and smooth, 1-3 second hold

PROGRESSION VARIABLES
No weights, add weights, 2 feet to 1 foot. I highly suggest not to use weights over 8 pounds

PROGRESSION 1

Stand with feet shoulder width apart and shoulder blades retracted. Turn thumbs up and raise arms up at 45 degrees or at 10 o'clock & 2 o'clock. As you raise your hands, squeeze the shoulder blades and don't let your thumbs go above your ear lobes.

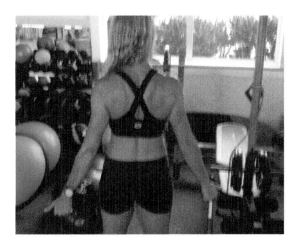 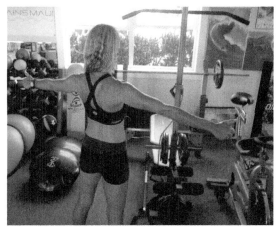

PROGRESSION 2

Add light (2-5 pound) weights, increase hold time

PROGRESSION 3

Stand on 1 leg

Exercise 4:
SELF MYOFASICAL RELEASE OF UPPER SHOULDER BLADES/UPPER BACK/LATS/QUADS/ADDUCTORS

Many people cringe at the sight of these rollers but I LOVE them. When you roll out the upper body muscles that help your shoulders move in sync, you reset the muscle pattern to its natural state. Rolling out various muscle groups also brings fresh blood to the muscles, allowing for faster recovery as it helps release harmful toxins that settle in.

In these exercises I am combining the areas of shoulder blades, upper back and latissimus dorsi. All of these muscles help the shoulders and upper body in maintaining better posture and range of motion, as well as helping the muscles of the shoulder perform better.

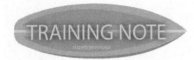

*A word of **CAUTION** regarding proper SMR Rolling:*

1. Avoid rolling "directly" on a sore or tender spot. This could cause more harm than good. If an area is already "inflamed" roll a few inches near it. Work your way towards the area but in an indirect, careful manner.

2. Slow down; don't roll too fast. If you roll too fast you won't get the benefits. Slowly prepare yourself for each part of the body as not to shock it. Let your brain and body get used to this feeling.

3. Don't spend too much time on one tender area. If you spend, say, 5 minutes that's way too long. You might think you're doing no harm but it's time to roll on. You could actually cause nerve or tissue damage. Spend 20 seconds per area, max.

4. NEVER roll out your lower back. It makes me crazy to see people do this because it's very dangerous. There are little bones in your lower back called spinal facets that you can actually fracture with your own weight. Stick to the upper back region.

5. Opinions have changed on the rolling of the IT Band and it is suggested to stretch it or use forms of ice therapy rather than rolling it. I will show you stretches for the IT Band in the next exercise.

SUGGESTED TRAINING EQUIPMENT
Firm or extra firm 36 inch long foam roller, also referred to as self myofascial roller

SUGGESTED REPS/SETS
Before and after each paddling session. Once you find a spot, hold for 20 seconds if possible.

PROGRESSION VARIABLES
Firmer roller

Shoulder Blades/Upper Back

Think of your shoulder blades as having many dimensions instead of just being flat. There are lots of layers of muscles that lay on top of each other that need rolling. This is great!

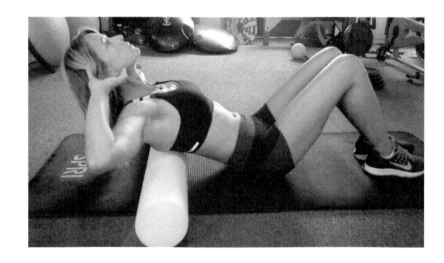

Lie on the floor with knees bent and hands behind your head. Do not clasp fingers together. Situate the foam roller horizontally across the upper region of your back so it is directly underneath the shoulder blades. Raise hips off the floor to apply more pressure. (See video mentioned earlier in this chapter.) Try to turn and change the angle of the roller on the shoulder blade to reach all pockets of muscle. If you find a sore spot, breathe through it and try to let the muscle release.

You might hear some popping; that's okay. That's just bubbles of gas releasing. Keep at it until the intensity of sensation you feel is lower.

Latissimus dorsi

Also referred to as "lats." These powerful muscles help the body flex and rotate, and assist you as you pull your body to the shaft of the paddle. They are prone to getting sore and tired.

Lay on your right side and place roller under your armpit with your right arm fully extended outward. Bend your left leg behind you to use help lift and apply extra pressure. Lift body and roll in various angles in order to reach all parts of muscle. Caution, this could be very uncomfortable. Find a spot or area, hold 20 seconds then switch to left side.

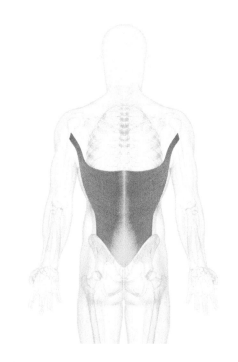

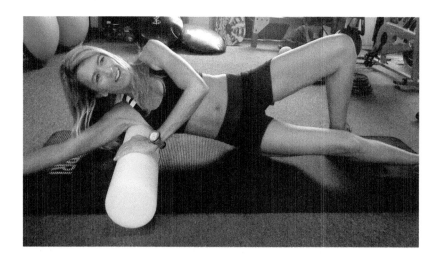

Quadriceps

Also referred to as thighs or quads. We roll out the quads to help the hip flexors release any pulling that may be happening. Pulling forward of the hip flexors can lead to lower back pain and the leg muscles also benefit.

Turn onto your stomach and place the roller horizontally across your upper thighs with your elbows supporting you (guys watch out for your package) and scoot yourself along the full thigh to the top of the knee. **CAUTION**: Do not roll on top of your knee cap. Do this a few times and see where you may be tender.

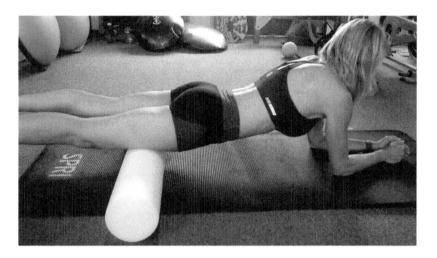

Adductors

Also referred to as inner thighs. These are usually weak and undertrained. By rolling this just a little, it will go a long way in your total functional performance.

You can roll right into this position from the above exercise by making like a "V" with your legs. Turn your feet outward or inward and you'll likely find some spots that could use a little love. Go easy.

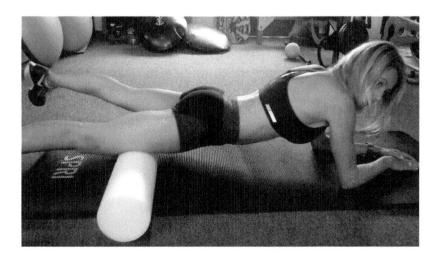

Exercise 5:
STRETCHES FOR THE IT BAND

Iliotibial band stretch: Standing
Cross one leg in front of the other leg and bend down and touch your toes. You can move your hands across the floor toward the front leg to you will feel more stretch on the outside of your thigh on the other side. Hold this position for 15 to 30 seconds. Return to the starting position. Repeat 3 times. Reverse the positions of your legs and repeat.

Iliotibial band stretch: Side-leaning
Stand sideways near a wall. Place one hand on the wall for support. Cross the leg farthest from the wall over the other leg, keeping the foot closest to the wall flat on the floor. Lean your hips into the wall. Hold the stretch for 15 seconds, repeat 3 times, and then switch legs and repeat the exercise another 3 times.

Standing calf stretch
Facing a wall, put your hands against the wall at about eye level. Keep one leg back with the heel on the floor, and the other leg forward. Turn your back foot slightly inward (as if you were pigeon-toed) as you slowly lean into the wall until you feel a stretch in the back of your calf. Hold for 15 to 30 seconds. Repeat 3 times and then switch the position of your legs and repeat the exercise 3 times. Do this several times each day.

Hamstring stretch on wall
Lie on your back with your buttocks close to a doorway, and extend your legs straight out in front of you along the floor. Raise one leg and rest it against the wall next to the door frame. Your other leg should extend through the doorway. You should feel a stretch in the back of your thigh. Hold this position for 15 to 30 seconds. Repeat 3 times and then switch legs and do the exercise again.

Quadriceps stretch
Stand an arm's length away from the wall with your injured leg farthest from the wall. Facing straight ahead, brace yourself by keeping one hand against the wall. With your other hand, grasp the ankle of your injured leg and pull your heel toward your buttocks. Don't arch or twist your back. Keep your knees together. Hold this stretch for 15 to 30 seconds.

Exercise 6:
FOREARM STRETCHES AND EXERCISES FOR PADDLER'S ELBOW

This helps treat that nagging tenderness and weakness right at the outside of the elbow where the lateral extensors connect and are prone to overuse. Refer to the earlier section of this chapter.

I've had to see a sports doc myself about this and said he gets lots of paddlers coming in for it, as well. He suggested icing area after training and/or paddling and performing the following stretches as often throughout the day as possible. I found that the icing was key.

SUGGESTED TRAINING EQUIPMENT
1-5 pound dumbbell

SUGGESTED REPS/SETS
Before and after each paddling session and throughout the day. At least 3-5 times for 20 seconds each side 1-2 times per day.

PROGRESSION VARIABLES
Once pain and inflammation is gone you can attempt a gentle strengthening exercise. Consult with your doctor.

While sitting or standing extend your right arm out in front of you and make a gentle fist. Take your left hand and cup the right hand and pull the hand towards you, hold for 20 seconds, release and repeat. You can relax your hand at this point as you continue to stretch with each rep.

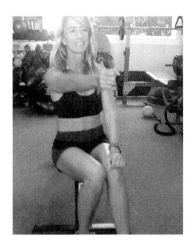 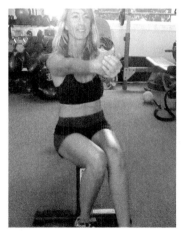

Once you're feeling a bit better, you can attempt to introduce a light strengthening exercise designed to strengthen the extensors.

Sit on a chair next to a table. Place a thin cushion or roll up a gym towel so your arm and wrist are supported, with your palm

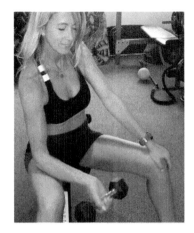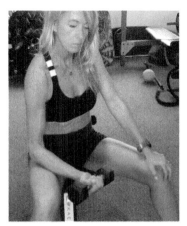

facing down. Take the weight in your hand and let the weight fall or roll toward the ground. You can do this 20-30 times. Consult your physician

Exercise 7:
CHEST OPENER ON SMR ROLL

As I mentioned earlier your posture as a stand up paddler will always be important and you will constantly need to be aware of it on and off the water. As you add more miles and strokes the larger stabilizing muscles of the chest will also need some help. The pectoral wall of the chest wall can be incredibly short and tight. This exercise will help you open up your chest, which will allow for better overall posture.

SUGGESTED TRAINING EQUIPMENT
Moderate to firm roller

SUGGESTED REPS/SETS
Before and after each session. As long as you like!

PROGRESSION VARIABLES
None

Place your foam roller lengthwise on the ground and sit on the end. As you lower your back and upper body along the length of the roller, knees bent, feet on the floor, tilt your pelvis forward. DO NOT allow your lower spine to have pressure in the sacral area. Your head must be fully supported by the roller.

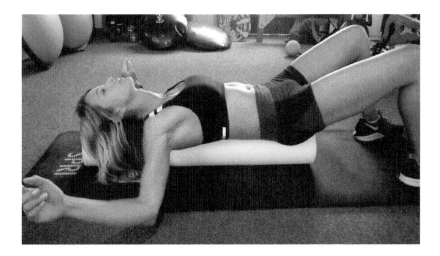

Open your arms and just let your arms fall with the backs of the hands facing the ground. Enjoy the stretch! Don't force anything; just let it go.

Exercise 8:
LOWER BACK STRENGTHENER - SIMPLE HAMSTRING STRETCH

When the lower back suffers, it's typically due to tighter muscles in other areas, such as the hamstring muscle, for one, from being over active, or from having a weak core. This simple hamstring stretch is just a reminder of how easy it is to help your lower back. After this section go back to Chapter 2 and revisit those exercises.

Lie on your back with your legs extended and your back straight. Keep your hips level and your lower back down on the floor. Bend your right knee towards your chest, keeping your left leg extended on the floor.

Slowly straighten your right knee, grabbing the back of your leg with both hands. While keeping both hips on the floor pull your leg toward you gently. Breathe deeply and hold for 10-30 seconds. Repeat on opposite side.

Stretch to the point of "mild discomfort," not to the point of pain. Never bounce. Keep your hips down on the mat. Try to keep the leg as straight as possible, only pulling it closer to you if your flexibility allows. To reduce the intensity of this stretch, bend the knee of the stretching leg.

RECOVERY AND THE IMPORTANCE OF REST

I would have to say that if there is one thing and one thing only that you take away from this book that would be this section right here. We paddle a lot of hard and long miles on the water and train and push to the max. If you find yourself out of whack and you're making bad decisions on race day, getting injured too much, or not feeling your best, maybe you just need to prioritize a few things in your life. Dare I say?

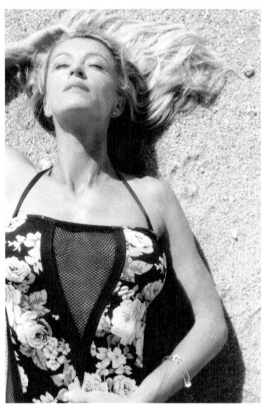

There have been so many athletes I've trained that have set themselves up for disappointment by not tapering down a bit better on their training or scheduling too many races that make them burn out early. They often get hurt because they weren't on top of their game.

photo by Tracy Leboe

If you're making lots of personal sacrifices and things start to unravel it's time you take a bit of an inner inventory to make things right. Don't forget that you've made a decision to be the kind of paddler you are, whether as a weekend warrior or by competing at pro level. Your friends and family already know that your time to train is important, but don't forget about them and how they support you. You get my drift?

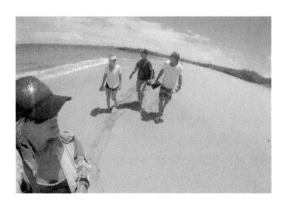

How to Increase Your Stand Up Paddling Performance

Here some basics to help you practice proper recovery so you have the most wins on the water and in life:

1. Plan your rest days. Just as you'd plan your training days, mark on the calendar scheduled rest days and guard them. This is when your body will make muscle repairs and allow for stress hormones, such as cortisol, to return to a normal state. Let your body rebuild and store up on the good things.

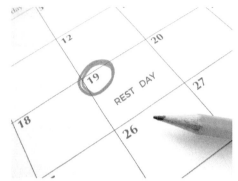

2. Get quality sleep. I often joke wish I could check into a hotel to get a good night's sleep. Consistently getting a good night's sleep will help glycogen stores rebuild more quickly and will also help stabilize important hormones that keep your mood steady.

Studies show that if you continually lack sleep and find yourself deprived of REM sleep, your performance could suffer.

3. Cross train. Your body and your mind need you to give it some rest to repair itself. Still, some of the best athletes in the world have a really hard time doing so. I often tell my clients to change gears—especially before a big event. Go for a mellow bike ride, run on the beach with a friend, kick a soccer ball around a big open field, and just get off the water to do something totally different.

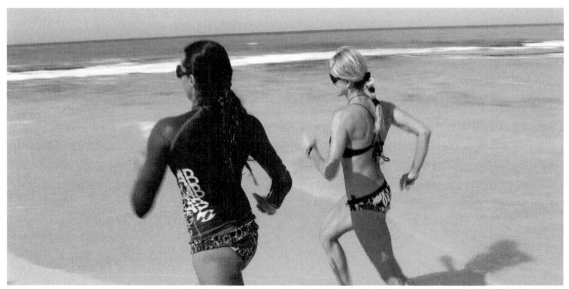

photo by Tracy Leboe

4. Pay attention to nutrition. You've worked so hard to perform so well, why stop now? Don't poison your paddling machine with junk. Watch the garbage and maintain your normal healthy routine. I will say you can reward yourself with one meal that makes you smile. You can pig out occasionally; just don't make a habit of it.

5. Hydrate. If you're going to celebrate, go easy. I'm not saying a tasty cold beer is bad, just maybe have one—not six. Be sure to up your water intake so you can bathe your body so that all your cells can heal. Refer back to Chapter 8 on selecting the right recovery drink.

I have a true story to share with you now. My personal doctor, an internist here on Maui named Rick Sands, is my good friend, mentor, and amazing paddling athlete. One day when I came to him about the ciguatera toxin I manage, I was a bit frustrated, and very down in the dumps about having to deal with it. This particular time I was worried about the M20 and how my health condition would be affected during and after the finish.

He took both of my hands and looked me in the eyes and said, "Suzie, I am giving you permission not to go so hard. I want you to give *yourself* permission not to go so hard." I looked at him as if he had three heads and then the tears came as I sank sobbing in his arms. It was like someone said it's okay to go easy.

No one in my life ever gave me permission to throttle back and "slow down." That's because I never allowed myself, until just a few years ago, to find a better balance.

As simple as that sounds, it really helped. I was overtraining and finding my training and performance getting flat and stale. He said again, "Suzie, I want you to give yourself permission not to go so hard. Do the race but don't go so hard." Thank you Rick! I'll never forget that.

I turned my focus and stress into a great finish and a great race day with my relay partner and good friend, Stephen Ross. I felt fresh and made peace with the fact that my health comes first. Luckily I felt so good that day I was able to push a bit harder—but not to the point of mental or physical failure. That day changed my life.

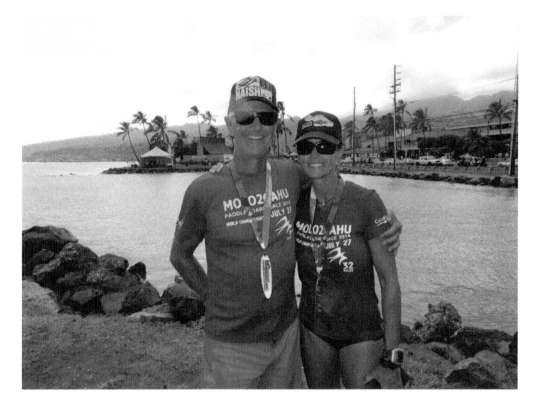

Follow these tips and I hope that you'll remain injury-free and paddling strong.

Now that you have a good idea on how to avoid common overuse injuries, next take a peek in the amazing world of downwind paddling. This is my passion. I hope that one day you can come to Maui and paddle Maliko with me!

CHAPTER 11
Training Tips for Downwind Paddling

- The lure of downwind paddling.
- Do you need to be a surfer?
- Downwind gear does matter.
- Bump hunting: reading the water, wind and more.
- The downwind paddle stroke versus flat water stroke.
- Strength training for downwind paddling.
- Cardio training for downwind paddling.
- Ocean safety and downwind paddling.

I've saved the best for last and have so much to share in this chapter. I am also stoked to bring you lots of great advice and knowledge from Jeremy Riggs, my downwind coach and Maui's own downwind champion.

Downwinding is, for sure, hands down my passion and favorite type of paddling. Downwind racing is my second favorite. I love it so much because it blends surfing with paddling for nonstop adrenaline. Whenever I'm downwind paddling I feel a constant surge of "Oh my God this is insane!" Here I'm paddling with Maliko sensation Graison Poledna from Seattle. He's only 11 years old! He was hanging tough with our large crew as gusts clocked over 40mph and wind and ground swells were running approximately up to 6 feet. He kept his head and cool and understands the importance of safety, thanks to his coach Jeremy Riggs.

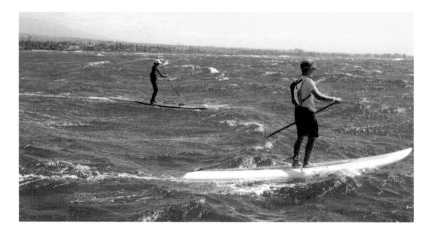

If you've thought about downwind paddling or dreamed of coming to Maui and doing our famous Maliko Run, then keep reading. It's definitely a different style of paddling and requires more skill and training then you might think.

All of the cool photos in the magazines really don't do downwind paddling justice. Unless you're the guy on the ski, photographing and getting the real perspective, it's hard to really grasp the enormity of it all. Speaking of perspective, here's a killer shot of Jeremy Riggs coming down a monster swell near Pier One. This is the real deal and not just a camera angle. THIS is what we live for. Super cool.

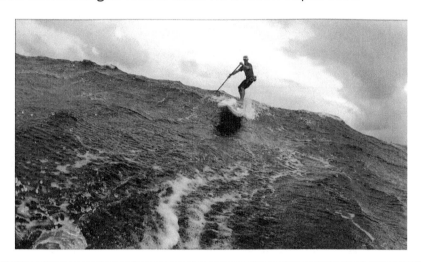

Jeremy Riggs *writes about why he loves downwind paddling: "There are so many reasons that I love downwind paddling. The first thing that got me into paddling with the wind was the feeling of surfing the wind swells. I love the feeling I get from the speeds we are able to reach on the bigger ocean swells. We're hitting 14-15mph on a good Maliko run. Downwind surfing also takes intense concentration on the water and swells around you. You don't have any time for anything else to enter your mind when you are in the zone and searching for the next bump or a connection to another bump. The things I work on the most during a downwind run is slowing down, being relaxed and trying to keep my eyes scanning the ocean surface so I know when to paddle and where to go with the bumps."*

The troughs are bigger in real life and the open ocean that surrounds you is so much bigger than a two page spread. There's also the shark element. Yes I said it. The man or woman in the striped suit, oh ya they surf too. In the shot below Loch Eggers is flying down the coast as Darrell Wong captures this great photo.

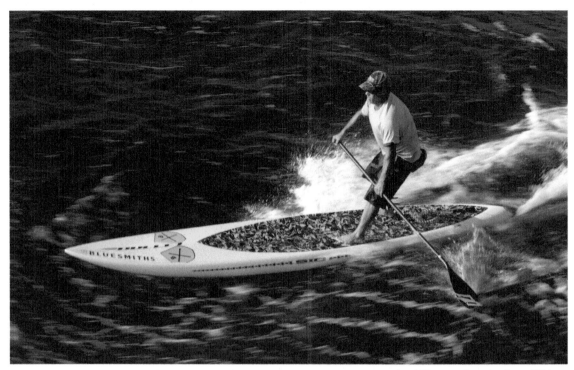

Loch Eggers photo by Darrell Wong

Not to scare you but yes, it's kind of big deal to go for a downwind paddle on Maui. You need to have a lot of water and ocean confidence, as well as knowledge about the weather, tides and surf heights in the area where you're paddling. From there it's pure water time and training in a very different way.

I've written a few articles about downwind paddling. During the OluKai Demo Day Training Session I hosted, I talked about how to be an all dimensional paddler. And that's what it takes; you have to be a multi-dimensional paddler to be successful on a downwind run. During a downwind you aren't just going fast and paddling in one direction. You are hunting, carving, and doing short cardio blasts of interval sprints to catch the best conveyor belt of bumps or glides that can last as long as 3 minutes.

Never have I had so much fun while paddling in comparison to riding a dirt bike and looking and hunting for the right jump, or seeking the angle of berm to pull into. While downwind paddling, your eyes are always gazing left to right and beyond, seeking the best opportunity for the ride of your life.

Not a surfer?

Well I would be lying if I didn't say it doesn't hurt to be a surfer or have some surf experience. The knowledge you get from surfing really goes a long way on a downwinder. I'm referring to surfing and not just paddle surfing. Downwind paddling, especially the Maliko Run and downwinding in the Pailolo Channel (which is between Maui and Molokai) is definitely for the advanced paddler.

Jeremy Riggs explains, "Paddlers with a surf background will have a little bit of a head start when it comes to footwork and understanding how to work with the rails of the board. Being able to stay balanced while riding swells and paddling in the ocean can make up for a lack of surfing experience. A good stable board is the best thing to have when you are learning to paddle downwind."

With combined wind swells and ground swells there are times when you might look down the nose of your board and think, "Holy crap, this is it! A freaking 7 foot drop!" That can go on for miles. You paddle, catch a bump, and take off. Then your friend next to disappears into the deep blue, down a trough of his or her own, appearing again later with a grin a mile wide.

> *Warning: resist the temptation to look behind you because you are guaranteed to mess in your board shorts or bikini bottoms!*

To prepare for the thrill I highly suggest you take a few surf lessons to really get the feel of a wave's energy and, more importantly, to learn how to find the sweetest part or the most powerful part of a wave. You will also benefit from learning about the wave's energy and how you will respond to it. This is almost like dancing.

Once you learn about the mechanics of a wave, you need to learn how to transfer your body's power and use the force of the wave to your biggest advantage. You don't just stand and go; you lean or bend or move your chest over your leg to get more board speed, or you lean back to avoid a pearling of the nose and to trim the board.

The waves don't need to be big during your lesson for you to benefit. They need to be just big enough so that you can watch the water moving in front of the nose of the board, to the side, and down the line. You'll learn how to maximize each ride and, in time, when to carve and turn to make it even a longer ride.

When taking a surf lesson, in addition to learning proper surf etiquette and courtesy, you'll get a natural feel for how the water moves under you and around you. You'll start to look at the ocean with a new pair of eyes. You'll notice if the wind is blowing off the tops of the waves, or if the water where you are is a weird formation like a churning bowl, if the sides or shape of the waves are more an "A" frame shaped or sharply peaked. You'll gain a different level of appreciation when you're watching patterns of the water moving and noticing how it responds to all the elements. So, for example if the swell or wave is more "A" framed shaped, it will be easier to surf as you're catching a big glide down the face of it versus a steep, more pitchy wave that may cause your board's nose to pearl.

Paddle surfing is also a great way to prepare yourself for downwind paddling. The footwork involved in surfing transfers right to your longer downwind board—but you'll take bigger steps. The comfort you have moving all over your paddle board in all kinds of conditions, including waves, big and small, will serve you well during your first downwinder.

However, all of this being said, don't be discouraged if you find yourself on Maui and you've never surfed or paddle surfed before you attempt your first downwinder. I urge you to go with someone well qualified so you have the best and safest experience.

DOWNWIND GEAR MAKES A DIFFERENCE

Like everything else we do in SUP, including training, your gear selection for downwind paddling is important, as are some of the accessories you can use to increase your performance. For example, you can have fun on a 12'6" board or on a 14ft board. There are also boards that are 16ft and longer with rudders to help you steer.

Shapes of the boards will vary but most that do well in downwind are really streamlined and made for "surf speed." However, others have shapes that allow you to punch through and exit fast: providing great stability without loss of speed. Tail shapes are also varied but those that are more along the lines of a surf shape (pulled in tail) may perform better. You want a tail to help you carve, maintain speed and then release you into the next bump. Do your homework here because, as like hems on skirts, they change and improve all the time.

Paddle selection can vary, depending on the board you're using. If you're stepping up to a longer board make sure you lengthen your paddle accordingly. I prefer a fixed carbon paddle but some people like the option of using an adjustable. Again, it's personal preference. Trends with paddles change and people move from super long paddles to those on the shorter side. Too tall and you might get some upper back pain, too short and your lower back may suffer. Try out what works best for you and make sure you have good stroke technique and super a strong core.

You need a leash to keep your board attached to you, but you do have leash options. Some people like the coil leashes and others the standard leash. I prefer the standard thin, straight leash so that if the board starts to spin in the direction of my head after a wipeout I have a little distance to avoid getting clocked pretty hard. Sometimes, however I will place a coil leash in the front loop of my rudder board that is used to place my paddle in when I carry the board.

Once you start getting faster and faster you may want to know exactly how fast you're going. Now you can track your speed live as a way to see how hard you are working or if you need to step it up.

If you missed it in chapter one titled, Gear Matters; I mentioned this new cool device called the Makai developed by Velocitek. It's GPS driven digital speedometer tool that you put on your downwind board. You can see in real time how fast you're going, how long you've been out and how far you've gone.

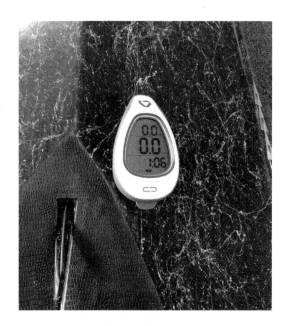

Jeremy Riggs loves it. Here's how he says the Makai can help you too: "The Makai speedometer by Velocitek is a great tool to have on your board while you are paddling. You can keep track of your speed during a run. Knowing that you have speed by glancing down is an immediate indication that you need to keep that speed up if you want to stay on that bump or find a new connection. You can also use the speed indications as a reminder that some of your poorly timed strokes are not yielding any increase in your speed. Cutting out some of these strokes will often allow the bumps to come to you quicker allowing you to position your board correctly to catch the next bump and it gives you a little more time to recover in between bumps."

DOWNWIND STROKE VERSUS FLAT WATER STROKE

This is really fun to talk about and yes, all of you technical stroke geeks could have forums just on this topic alone. The downwind paddling stroke is for sure unique but similar to that of other types of paddling. I'd have to say that it takes a bit more time finding a rhythm because there is usually more water moving around the blade and the conditions are constantly changing every few feet. The water is constantly moving, rising, and shifting. You also have a longer board, which means you have to reach farther during your stroke.

Jermey Riggs talks about the downwind stroke, saying, "The paddle stroke for downwind paddling and flat water paddling are very similar. You want a clean catch, powerful stroke and a timely exit. The technique is the same most of the time but the cadence and power output will change for downwind paddling. Your stroke needs to be timed perfectly with the passing swells to catch glides efficiently. You can paddle at a steady beat in flat water with the same intensity in every stroke. The power that you put into a stroke can vary when paddling downwind to match the speed of the swells you are catching and riding. "

I'd also like to add that when you're catching bumps, your first few strokes can be pretty explosive, but as you are actually gliding you might only be taking some light strokes to keep the board moving into the next bump. Watch some of Jeremy's videos on this. He makes it all look so easy!

Bump Hunting: Reading the water, wind and more

Let the downwind hunt begin. As I mentioned earlier, your eyes are the gateway to your next bump or glide. Once you've got one and are riding it you will constantly be looking for the next one to connect. It's like a fun game to me. Be careful, it is addicting.

There is definitely an art to being a great bump hunter. It takes time on the water, as well as many other skills, including knowing when it's prime downwind weather, understanding water conditions, and more.

Here's Jeremy Riggs' advice to those getting started in downwind paddling. "Start out in light wind and work up to the windier days. Learning to catch the smaller bumps on a light wind day will help tremendously when you are out on the windier days. On the windier days don't focus on catching the larger bumps."

"Keep your focus on the smaller and medium sized bumps and the bigger ones will then become much easier to catch. Try to maintain good posture while paddling and remember to stay relaxed and control your breathing. Get out there as much as you can. Your confidence will increase with each run, allowing you to focus more clearly and develop new skills."

People make the mistake of thinking that the bump they should catch is the one that they are paddling on or underneath them. The bump actually starts to form as the nose of your board enters the nice smooth area or "trough" in front of it. You will see a small ramp rising a bit bigger as you move forward. Just when you start to see an actual sort of line forming at the top of this ramp is when you need to hit it! That will be your next juicy glide! When you get a few in a row that form automatically, you've struck gold. Below is an example of what that sweet spot of the golden bump looks like:

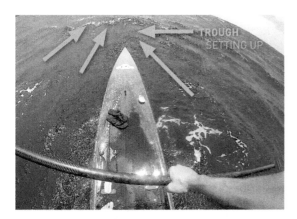
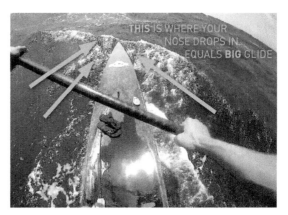

Another element to watch in downwind paddling is the wind. It's fun to watch it as it touches and flows across the water near you and in front of you. I've been a windsurfer all my life so reading the wind comes naturally to me. I used to brace myself when I could see a squall forming and heading towards me. That meant I would need to hold on tight. In downwind paddling you can't tell when a gust is coming because you actually feel it on your back! It's a rush. If you're not used to high winds hitting your body it's a bit unnerving at first. You will learn to love it.

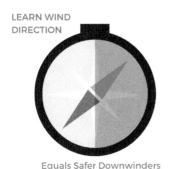

LEARN WIND DIRECTION

Equals Safer Downwinders

You can get used to the wind on your back, side of your cheek, or body. Try and figure out what direction it's coming from because that totally affects the amount of energy you'll need to spend and in what direction. If the wind shifts from perfect downwind to on or offshore you better get ready to work harder because it will be pushing you right or left instead of straight.

I've had a few days doing a Maliko run and it's like that song "smoke on the water." I doubt the band members of Deep Purple had that in mind.

Look at cloud formations before and while you're paddling. Changes in cloud formations can signal that more wind is coming or that the wind could be dying. I've lived on Maui now for 16 years and, as a windsurfer I've been learning all there is to know about trade wind clouds. Clouds that usually sit high above the West Maui mountains are a good sign, called altocumulus standing lenticularis, also affectionately called "lennies" clouds.

See what you learn reading this book?

When you see a huge, thick cloud bank (I'm talking about Maui here), usually on the front of that shear-like cloud is A LOT of wind that is gusty with trade showers. Those are fine. What's not fine is when that big mass follows you down the coast and shuts down your wind, and sometimes your vision too. We've had days where that horizontal wind shear shows itself on top of us with lots of rain. It gets violent sometimes. These squalls often pass through. At the time you will notice that the wind direction of that shear can seem like it's coming at you from all directions.

Finally, learn all you can about tides, wind swell and ground swell. The heights, of tides low or high, can have an effect on the wave and/or swell height.

Kahului Tide Prediction		
01:04 AM	Low Tide	0.27 foot
01:23 PM	Low Tide	1.21 foot
06:33 PM	High Tide	1.63 foot
08:15 AM	High Tide	1.65 foot

All of these elements also play a huge factor especially on the Maliko Run. The seasons and time of year will dictate when and where there is large, big surf and swell, so be mindful when you plan your trip to Maui.

Typically the winter swells starting arriving end of November and can last through May. Ideally, June through September will be a better time to do a downwinder here.

No matter where you may seek to paddle a downwinder, find out as much local knowledge as possible before going.

The more you know about weather the more success you will have about picking the good and safe days to downwind paddle.

STRENGTH TRAINING FOR DOWNWIND PADDLING

In addition to maybe taking a few surf lessons or getting lots more practice on your paddle surfboard to get your wave knowledge and footwork moving, you will also need to do downwind-specific strength training.

You need combined strength in your **core, upper body**, and, really, **your legs and your mind**. Some clients I've taken on a Maliko run are shocked to discover how tired their legs are from working the whole length of the board or from learning the different stance changes that are constant. It takes more leg endurance than you might think. Also note—your stroke will vary in length and in intensity depending upon conditions.

Then as I've mentioned earlier in Chapter 6, downwind paddling requires a strong heart because of all of the short cardio blasts and interval sprints you will perform during the span of a few strokes.

You can also refer to my article on Cardio Training for Downwind Paddling here *http://bit.ly/1LVQdFl*

LEGS

So first, lets talk **legs**. Your legs act like pumps that help you drive power from your hips to the board. Then they help maintain balance and speed through the bump. You put them to use when walking forward or back along the board to position yourself better to catch the bump. There is a series of position changes the legs are constantly making in a repetitive manner.

1. Driving power through hips to legs.

2. Being sharp and consistent with balance.

3. Stepping back to surf stance position.

4. Stepping back towards the handle to repeat the process.

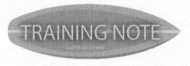

Your legs need endurance, balance training, and strength to help you squat low then recoil back up and to move forward toward the handle again. Definitely check out the exercises from Chapters 3 on balance and Chapter 5 on legs. Really try to perform some of the balance challenge progressions to fatigue. Feel the burn just enough, and each time you do, think of one more bump or glide you just caught!

Jeremy Riggs adds, "Having strong legs is important for both downwind and flat water but you will need to be more agile and quick on your feet to keep the board running smooth and stable during a downwind run. Balance is the key."

You can never get enough balance training, especially for downwind paddling. You can also juice up the legs a bit with more squats and lunges. Maybe sprinkle in the split jump lunges that are explosive and will give you that vision of come up from your big swell drop and down again.

CORE

Next we'll talk about your **core**. You should be an expert on this by now and realize that using your core is how you begin the driving of your hips, transferring energy to your legs to the board, which helps create momentum through the water. Remember, your paddle is secondary and acts as a guide.

Refer back to Chapter 2 on the core, which will give you tons of exercises to progress through. Some of my favorites that come to mind are the **10 & 2's** with the stability ball between your legs and the one where you balance on the stability ball with your knees with an 8 pound medicine ball or dumbbell, moving the ball toward you and away from you.

All core work is awesome—just understand the relationship of the work to paddling and try to visualize all of the anatomical points of your body as you begin each downwind paddling stroke to transfer that power.

UPPER BODY

And last, the **upper body**. I'd say here you can turn on the heat a bit more with emphasis on your chest, deltoids and upper back with more reps for endurance. You don't need a huge amount of weight. It's all about endurance and smooth, fast, power strokes.

The first exercise that comes to mind to me are the shoulder **tube chops** in Chapter 5 under "shoulder." These really bring it all together and target not only the shoulders but also the lats and chest pectoral wall that helps you drive that paddle hard and deep. Your upper back, traps, and rhomboids serve to stabilize you while you paddle. Second choice would be the **1-armed medicine** or **BOSU push ups** that totally isolate the pectoral wall. Remember you can do those standard or with knees bent.

Then, of course, as I mentioned earlier, you also need time on the water. Putting together everything you've read here takes some time and a different way of thinking. You've got the ocean that's always giving and pushing back. There are some days you might think you're paddling in glue and that's because of currents and tides—not because of you. So don't get discouraged.

MIND

As I've mentioned earlier and illustrated, the "no ego" rule really applies here. Common sense must be first and there is no shame in doing smaller, mini downwinders first. Make sure your mind is clear and not full of fear because that will work against you and could cost you your life or someone else's.

You can always go another time when you're in s better head-space. Don't feel pressure if you think conditions are over your head, literally and mentally. If you step off the shuttle, especially with our crew at Maliko, it's okay not to go. We'd all rather not rescue you or put others in danger.

It's way more fun to have a great experience than a bad one, trust me.

OCEAN SAFETY AND DOWNWIND PADDLING:

I would be a horrible trainer if I didn't close here and talk a little bit about ocean safety and downwind paddling. This applies for anyone thinking about trying no matter where you live in the world.

A few tips

1. Always go with an experienced professional or friend who will be mindful of your well-being and theirs. I know lots of pretty serious water athletes who come to Maui and just do it because it's easy and no big deal. The last thing you want is to end up on the rocks and get cut or smashed by big waves. Having someone with local knowledge helps too.

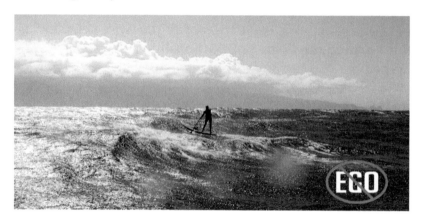

2. Really take inventory of your skillset. I can't tell you how important it is to leave your ego at the beach. And I can't tell you how many times people have talked themselves up to me only to be humbled pretty quick by my pre-downwind test. Not to pop your downwind paddling dream bubble, but be aware that you don't want to be a danger to yourself or to the person who is taking you. Do it in smaller steps and maybe go earlier in the day when the wind is usually lighter (unless it's the Gorge!). If there's surf, maybe pass until it comes down. And then maybe just go a few miles versus the longer distance and get your head on straight. You want to have a good experience not a life event!

3. Check your gear and check your gear. Always check the little string on the back of your board that ties your leash on and holds it all together. I keep 4 or 5 in my truck at all times and freely give them away. It can save your life. As a backup you can also use a zip-tie. If your board has a vent plug, make sure it's locked tight. Check the integrity of your leash. I know friends that double up on the super big days.

4. Don't be a hydration phobe because you think you won't look cool. Take some dang fluids with you. You have no idea what could happen. Maybe your friend will end up having an episode, in which case you will wish you had some water with you. There are so many small and comfortable hydration packs. For under an hour and a half on the water, water's fine to take. For paddling over an hour add a dash of electrolytes.

5. You may think it's overkill, but I always take my phone. I have actually had to call for help once when a buddy of mine's leash was spilt in half by a huge rogue set. It was a horrible day and I thought he died. As a step up, I also always have a satellite unit or beacon. We've had some big rough days and anything can happen. If a friend hits his or her head, there's a shark attack, or experiences any other life-threatening event, you'll be glad you have one.

6. Paddle with a buddy. I am so guilty of this. There are times when I have an unusual break in my day and no one is around. Sure there's peeps on the shuttle but when they're Dave Kalama or Kody Kerbox, they ain't waitin' for me. Even on the mellowest days I've had moments where I thought I saw something (tiger shark) or I had a weird fall or the wind dies. You just never know what might happen. It's one thing to tell someone you're out there but better to pair up for the paddle.

7. Last but not least, wear super bright neon clothing—a hat, a top, or both. The ocean is big and it's good for you to be seen by your buddy and others. Also, elements can change and that's why I love my BLUESMITHS top. It's real ocean performance paddling gear. I highly suggest you check them out.

*****

Well, you've come to the end of my book and I hope that you're stronger and ready to rock it out there. I would so love to hear how you're doing and encourage your emails or tags on Facebook.

Stand up paddling has offered me many life lessons and continues to make me push myself everyday. Being on the ocean often makes me feel like a speck of sand—especially during channel crossings. This photo was taken of me coming into the finish at the Maui to Molokai, 27 miles.

Conditions were less than ideal and I experienced stomach pain for 10 miles. However, the channel, like the M20, taught me so much about how much I don't know. I guess that's why I will keep going back.

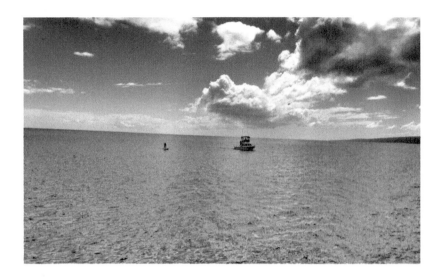

Should you like a personal consult but you live in Australia or New Zealand or Georgia, SKYPE is a blast and great way to connect. It's amazing what technology can do for your SUP performance.

And lastly, if you'd so be inclined, please write a review for me on Amazon!

Thank you sincerely for your friendship and sharing the stoke of SUP. Together, let's keep this amazing sport special where everyone feels welcome and encouraged to be the best human being they can be on and off the water.

Mahalo,

Suzie Cooney
Suzie Trains Maui

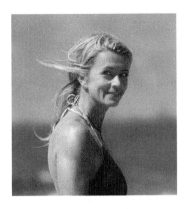

Meet Suzie Cooney

Personal Trainer, Professional Ocean SUP Athlete, Spokesperson, Sup Coach, SUP Event Director, Lifestyle & Sports Model

Suzie Cooney is known as one of the early female pioneers in stand up paddling. She is a sponsored ocean SUP athlete, a global figure and fitness authority for the sport of stand up paddling from its early development in 2008 and has been writing articles for books, magazines, and her personal blog.

She became passionate about SUP when she had an unusual accident in April of 2009, during which she broke her left leg and ankle and right ankle, leaving her in a wheelchair for over two months and on crutches for two more. She discovered stand up paddling was the best form of personal rehab.

Her mission became to tell the world to not to give up and to STAND UP. She created the world's first largest SUP event "STAND UP For Women's Health & Fitness," in January 2010, along with the Four Seasons; which attracted over 430 women from around the world.

From there she became ATHLETA's first SUP ambassador, is OluKai's Premium Footwear Annual Spokesperson for the Downwind Race Ho'olaule'a, Nominee for SUP Female Paddler of the year since 2012, and is also known for her passion of coaching and preparing new paddlers for downwinders on Maliko.

Her former years were spent windsurfing and completing motocross races as an adrenaline junkie. She admits that downwind paddling tops off her tank off nicely. Downwind paddling is definitely her passion and focus on Maui, but she also loves to paddle surf.

From a 7 year background in orthopedics sports medicine and surgery and, as a trainer for 13 years, she is able to fine-tune her clients on and off the water. She feels her client's body mechanics and power are as equally important as is the board under their feet. With all of these combined skills and experience, she likes to instill body, board, and ocean confidence.

Clients SKYPE train with her from around the world in preparation for their big debut on Maliko and for other SUP strengthening needs. Some train for channel crossings and others simply to enjoy the sport more or use SUP as a cross-training element for other sports.

"Suzie Cooney combines imagination, inspiration and perspiration. She's a one-of-a-kind waterwoman; a brilliant and patient teacher. Oh, and she is also a complete badass, which is the highest compliment I can possibly give." —Susan Casey, bestselling author of The Wave and previous editor in chief of *O, The Oprah Magazine* and *Outside magazine*.

Accomplishments

- Maui to Molokai 2015: solo 27 miles
- OluKai Downwind Race 2015: 1st Place Divisional
- Molokai 2 Oahu SUP Channel Crossing 2014: 32 miles, 5th in Relay Division
- Maui Paddleboard Championships 2013: 2nd, 14ft Age Division
- OluKai Hololaule'a 2011: 1st place,14ft Age Division
- Olukai Ho'olaulea Maliko SUP Race 2011: 1st place Age Division
- Naish International Championships Maliko SUP Race 2011: 6th place in Age Division.
- Created World's First & Largest International SUP Event in January 2010 with Four Seasons Maui: See News Coverage & Video
- OluKai Ho'olaule'a 2010: 3rd place, 14ft Age Division
- ATHLETA First Featured SUP Athlete 2010

Suzie also lives with the debilitating toxin called ciguatera poisoning since 2011, which is a constant battle and is triggered by the sun and intense or regular exercise. Stay tuned for a television special documentary to air this fall on Animal Planet. Learn more about ciguatera and discover how Suzie must cope with this condition for the rest of her life.

She is also an advocate for mental health as her mother lives with schizophrenia. She supports and is supported by Glenn Close' foundation, Bring Change 2 Mind.

To learn more about Suzie Cooney you can visit her website at *SuzieTrainsMaui.com*

Surf
- FB mates
- Boards Alaska, mike, Kyle, cruz, Jake
- ✓ Surf
PPlanner
- Plan

VB?
Verizon

Email JD
Call Jen, Nana, Kyle, ma youngs, Jake Blair

Saturd or Sunday Amigos

File Lost & Found
Babylon to Penn
1:52 pm → 3ish

Rebel Souljaz April 8

CPSIA information can be obtained at www.ICGtesting.com
Printed in the USA
BVOW07s1918180116

432980BV00015B/15/P